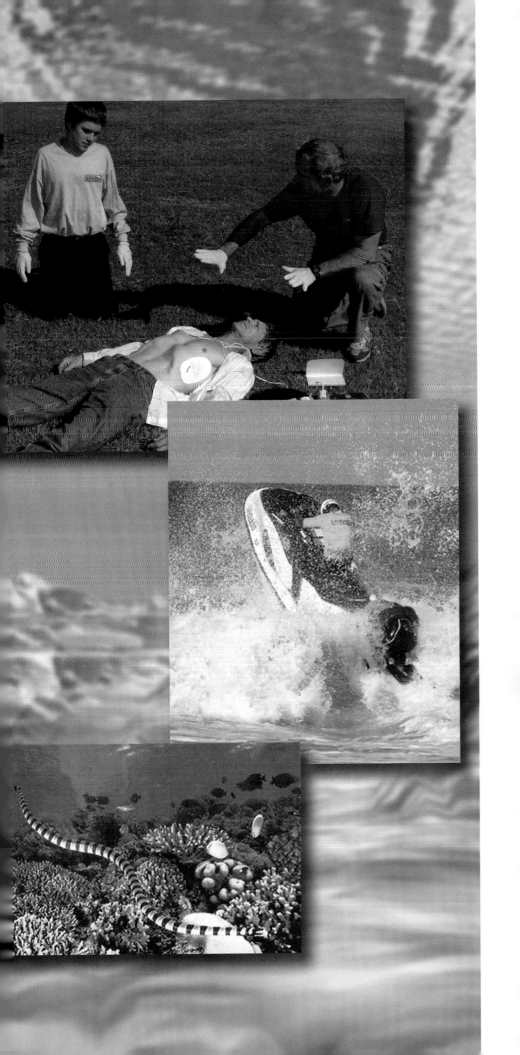

NAUI First Aid

Also Includes: CPR, Emergency Oxygen Administration, AED, Blood-borne Pathogens, and Aquatic Life Injuries First Aid.

PUBLISHED BY
National Association of Underwater Instructors, Inc. (NAUI)

PRODUCT DEVELOPMENT
Jed Livingstone

PRINCIPAL AUTHORS
Susan Carroll-Hamblen

EDITORS
Jed Livingstone and Peter Oliver

REVIEWERS
Dr. Ron Bangasser
Dr. Jolie Bookspan
Keith Sliman

DESIGN AND LAYOUT
Dennis Guzman Design

PHOTOGRAPHY
Scott Raish
Daniel Cullinane
Jed Livingstone
Peter Oliver
Wayne Hasson
Doug Shick
Neil Winkelmann
Daniel Morris, www.danielxmorris.com
Mike Carter, Beeline Photography, www.mikes2cents.com
Burt Jones and Maurine Shimlock, Field Museum of Natural History, www.fieldmuseum.org/aquaticsnakes
Joseph Berger, www.insectimages.org
Dave Powell and Arnold T. Drooz, USDA Forest Service, www.insectimages.org
James Gathany, John Wilson, Savannah River Ecology Laboratory, Centers for Disease Control and Prevention Public Health Image Library, http://phil.cdc.gov/phil/home.asp

Printed in the United States of America, Europe and the Pacific Rim

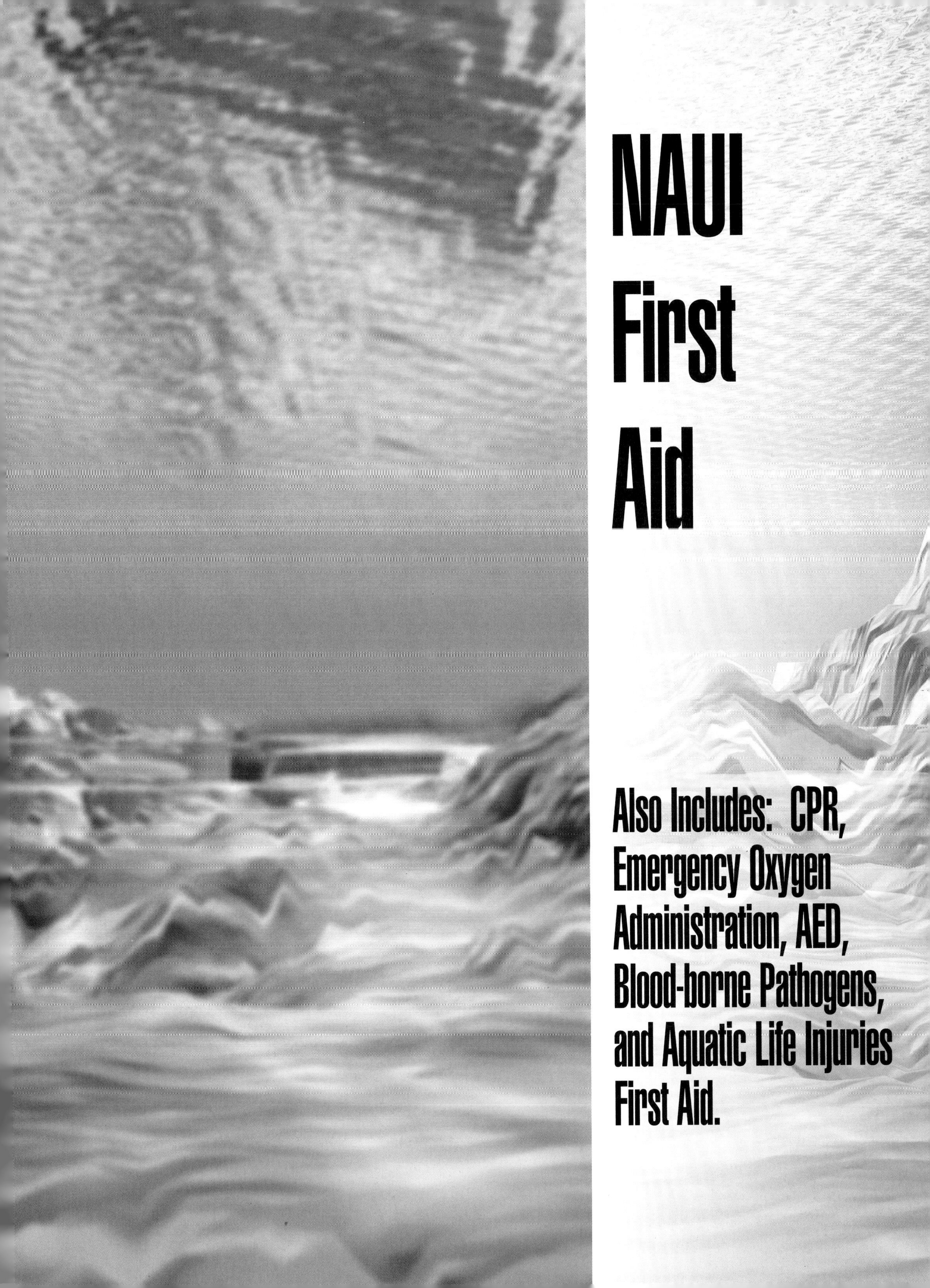

NAUI First Aid

Also Includes: CPR, Emergency Oxygen Administration, AED, Blood-borne Pathogens, and Aquatic Life Injuries First Aid.

PREFACE

First Aid and CPR for NAUI Divers and Leaders is a reference text and workbook for the NAUI First Aid, Cardio-Pulmonary Resuscitation (CPR), Emergency Oxygen Administration, Automated External Defibrillation (AED), and Blood-Borne Pathogen certifications available from NAUI. This text and its companion instructor guide conforms to the US Occupational Health and Safety Administration (OSHA) requirements for training in first aid and CPR, and incorporates the recommendations of the 2005 International Consensus Conference on Cardiopulmonary Resuscitation and Emergency Cardiovascular Care Science With Treatment Recommendations (CoSTR), hosted by the American Heart Association (AHA)in Dallas, Texas, January 23–30, 2005 and published concurrently in November 2005 in Currents (AHA) and Resuscitation (Elsevier, B.V.) magazines. Subsequently, the AHA and the European Resuscitation Council (ERC) published new guidelines incorporating the same recommendations for their respective courses and programs. This text and instructor guide is also consistent with those guidelines.

Since its inception in 1959 NAUI has required that candidates for membership – graduates of Skin Diving Instructor (SDI), Assistant Instructor (AI), Divemaster (DM), and Instructor courses – demonstrate competency in first aid and CPR skills as a prerequisite to membership in the Association. As underwater educators NAUI Instructors are also required to teach these skills to their diving students and to the general public. In the past NAUI as an association has either relied on or allied with other organizations to provide this training to our potential members. For some time, we have considered bringing the teaching of first aid and CPR "in-house." With the publication of this work, NAUI members now have NAUI approved course materials with which they will be able to train and qualify to teach these courses within their relevant professional capacities as SDI, AI, DM or Instructors

It is also important to note that as professional educators and aquatic experts, NAUI members are categorized similarly to lifeguards and other health care providers. As such, the level of training needed has been variously referred to in the past as "professional rescuer" or "CPR for the professional" and was useful to distinguish between those who needed to learn two-rescuer and infant-child CPR, rather than simple one-rescuer CPR for adults only. The latter was also referred to historically as "lay person" CPR.

NAUI divers, as opposed to NAUI leaders and instructors, are considered non-professional "lay" rescuers when providing first aid and CPR. However, unlike the general population, and because of their choice to become certified divers, they will find themselves in remote and exotic locations where EMS systems are primitive or non-existent. They will also confront first aid and rescue situations that will demand knowledge not typical of the general public or typical "lay" first aid provider. Therefore, and consistent with the 2005 Consensus Conference recommendations that training be tailored to meet the needs of the students, NAUI recommends that NAUI divers learn the additional content for providing "health care provider" level CPR skills to include two-rescuer, and infant-child CPR variations as well as diving-specific first aid procedures and competencies in AED, blood-borne pathogens, and oxygen administration. This is not to imply that this level of training is required in order to be certified as a NAUI Scuba Diver or any other non-leadership level NAUI certification course. As stated previously, this level of training has always been required for NAUI leaders and instructors.

This text and the instructor guide will also support CPR and first aid training courses for the general public. NAUI members who are authorized to teach NAUI First Aid and CPR and the ancillary topics of AED, Blood-borne Pathogens, and Emergency Oxygen Administration may register their graduating students with NAUI and deliver the appropriate NAUI certification cards and recognition materials. The specialized content recommended for NAUI divers and described in the previous paragraph should be omitted in courses delivered to this population in order to remain consistent with the 2005 Consensus Conference recommendations. More detailed information on course variations for differing audiences is presented in the instructor guide.

This text was critically reviewed by several healthcare professionals, including a physician, a physiological researcher, and an emergency medical technician. We wish to thank:

Dr. Ronald P. Bangasser, past president of the California Medical Association, board member of the Underwater Hyperbaric Medical Society, and director of the Wound Care Clinic at Redlands Community Hospital.

Dr. Jolie Bookspan, research physiologist, university and military laboratory research in human performance in normal to extreme environments (subaquatic, aviation, thermal, terrestrial, forensic) for acute and extended durations. University professor of anatomy and physiology, environmental physiology, exercise physiology, statistics, orthopedic and pain rehabilitation.

Keith Sliman, Director of Safety at Ford, Bacon and Davis, Inc., Emergency Medical Technician, current board member and past Chairman of the National Association of Underwater Instructors, and current board member of the Safety Council in Baton Rouge.

GETTING THE MOST OUT OF THIS BOOK

Throughout this study book there will be sections that require your special attention. The following icons are used to mark these sections.

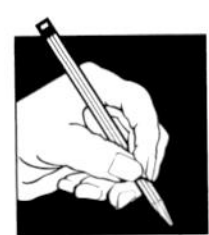

Indicates that you should take note of the information, it will help you complete the chapter review questions and it forms the basis for the final exam.

DEDICATION

NAUI First Aid is dedicated to Dr. Ron Bangasser, M.D. (1950-2007). Ron was a dear friend to NAUI and a tireless, enthusiastic, and positive force regardless of the subject that drew his attention. We were fortunate that he was able to serve as one of the reviewers of this work. That the resulting text is exemplary of NAUI's reputation for quality is due in no small part to his remarkable expertise and willingness to help. The world is a better place and diving is safer because of the example he set for all who knew him.

TABLE OF CONTENTS

Table of Contents

10 CHAPTER Shock 94

11 CHAPTER Soft Tissue Injuries 98

12 CHAPTER Musculoskeletal Injuries 106

13 CHAPTER Poisoning, Stings, and Bites 118

14 CHAPTER Other Medical Emergencies 128

15 CHAPTER Burns 136

16 CHAPTER Heat and Cold Emergencies 142

17 CHAPTER Water Hazards 148

18 CHAPTER Moving and Transporting Victims 170

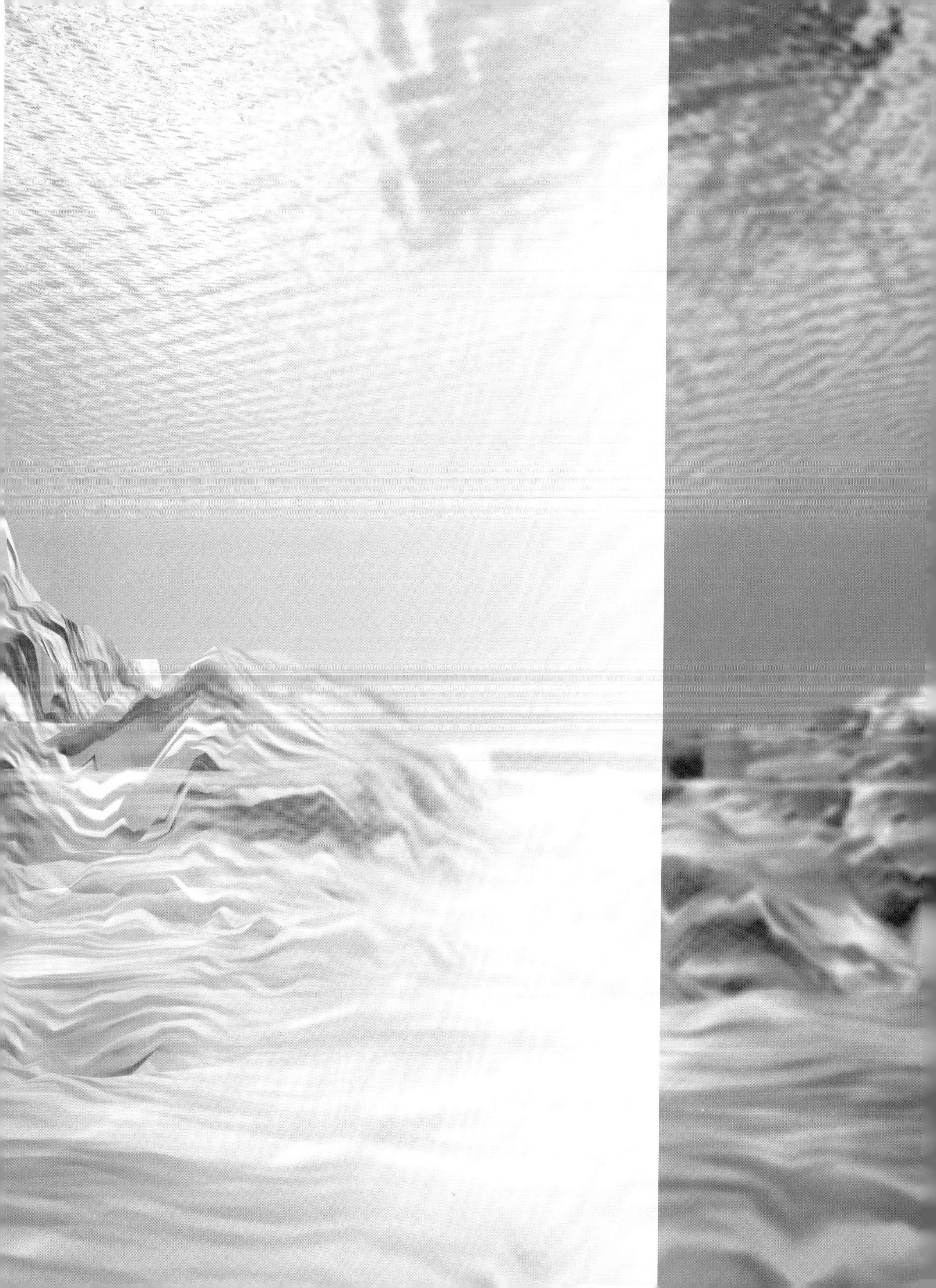

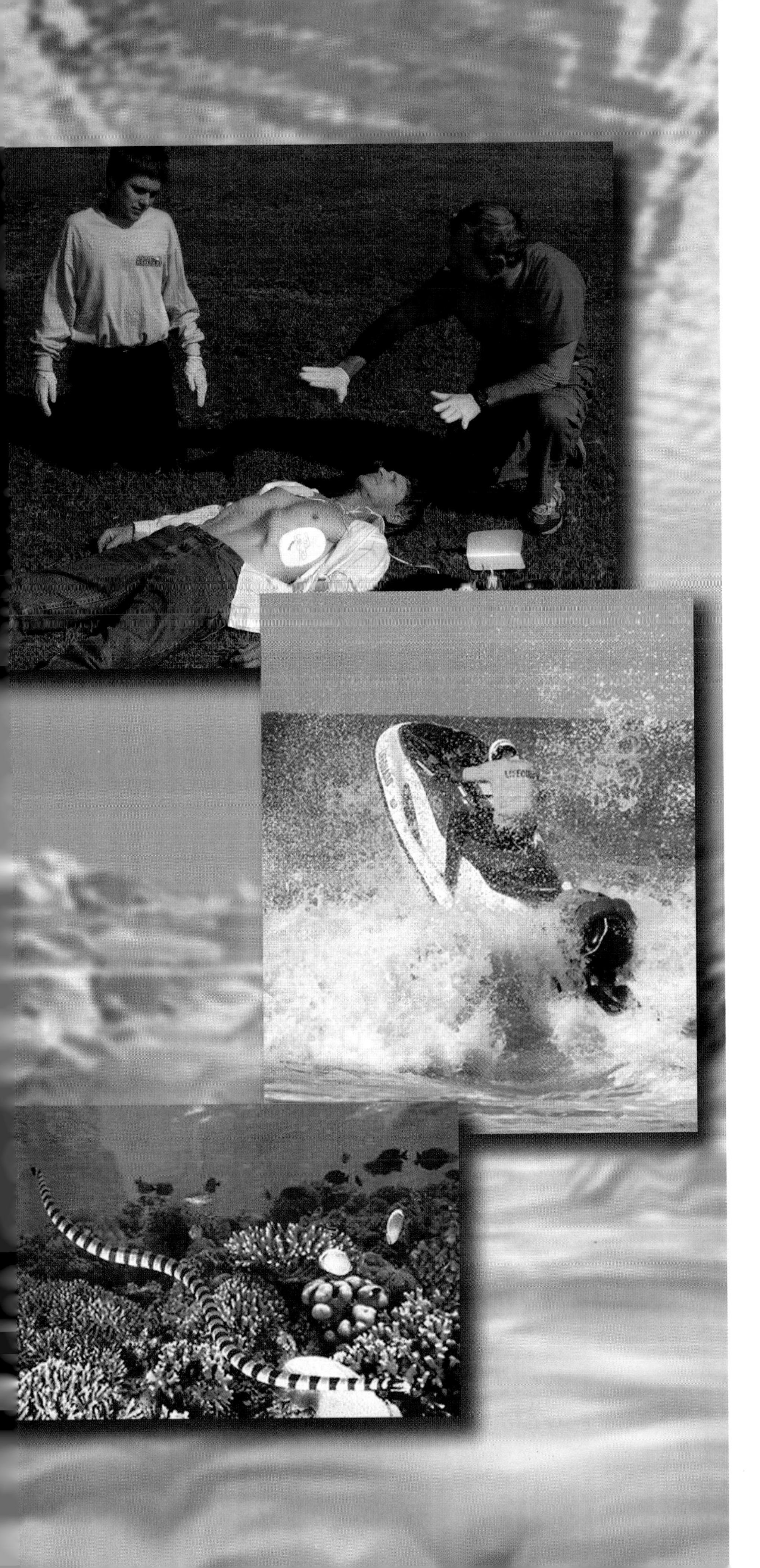

NAUI First Aid

Also Includes: CPR, Emergency Oxygen Administration, AED, Blood-borne Pathogens, and Aquatic Life Injuries First Aid.

CHAPTER 1 Introduction

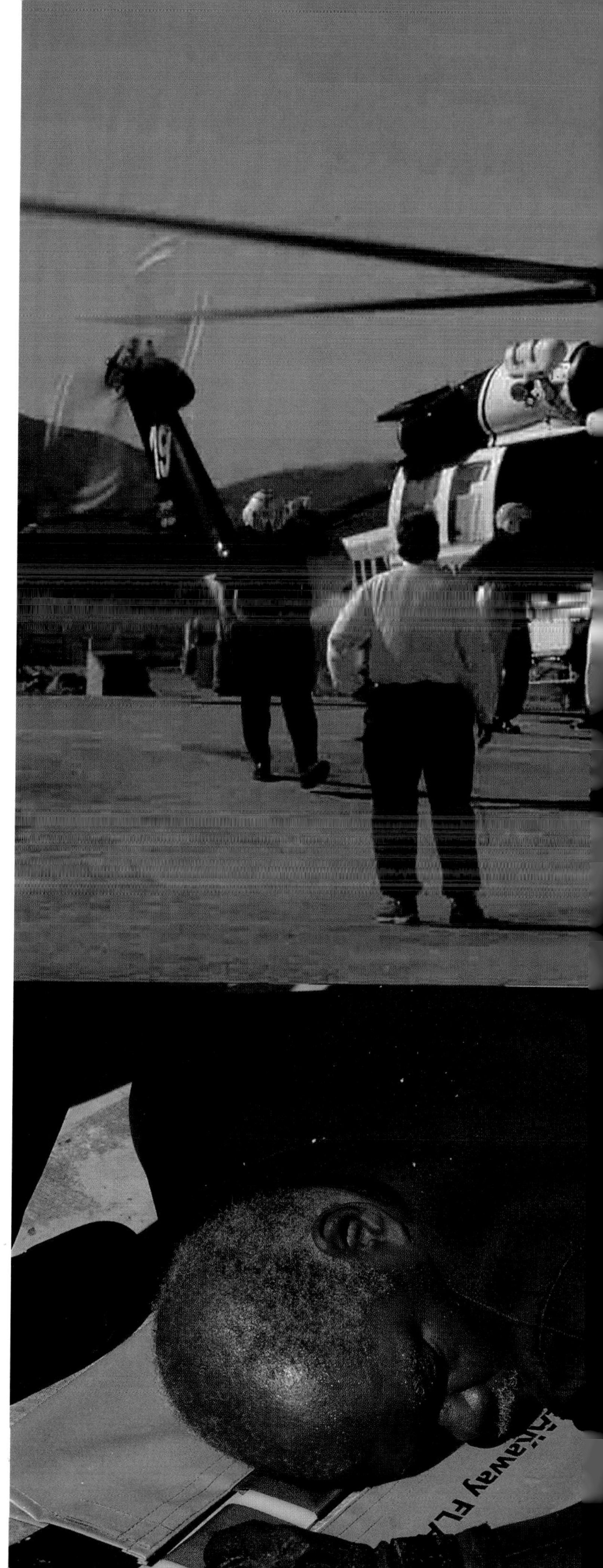

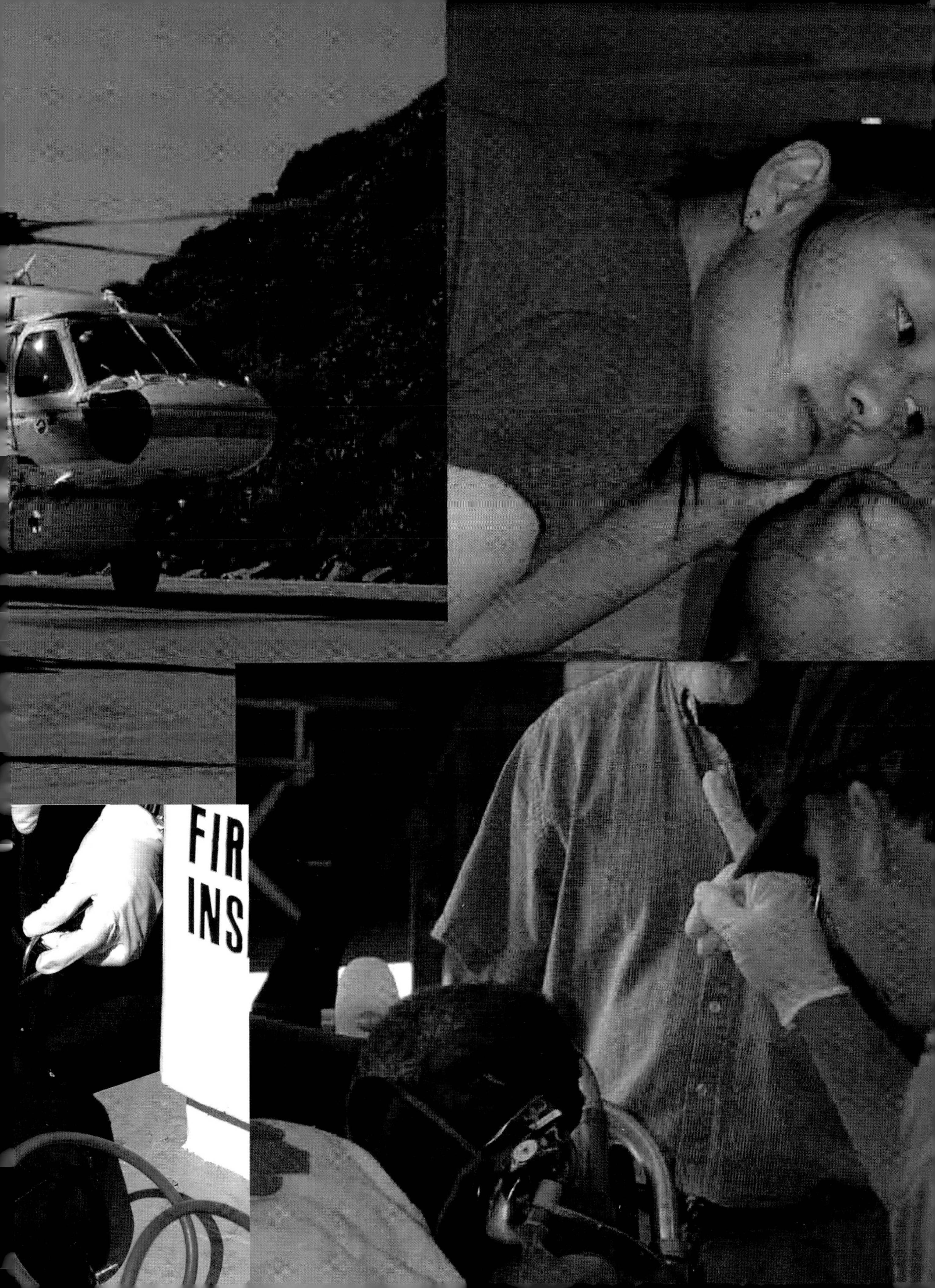
FIR
INS

Congratulations on your decision to take the NAUI First Aid course. You will find this to be a rewarding course, which will enable you to assist with emergencies whether they occur on a diving excursion or at home.

Accidents can happen anywhere, at any time, to anyone. Someday you might be called upon to aid a relative, friend, coworker, or even a complete stranger. Knowing first aid and the appropriate actions to take could save that person's life. This course will prepare you to know the steps to follow in an emergency, to aid the person in distress until they are in the care of medical personnel.

COURSE LEARNING GOALS

In this course you will learn about:

- Blood-borne pathogens
- Victim assessment
- Basic life support
- Adjunct life support
- Bleeding and shock
- Injuries and wounds
- Medical emergencies, such as poisoning, heart disease and stroke
- Environmental emergencies including: burns, heat and cold, water hazards, scuba diving maladies and aquatic life injuries
- Victim handling

COURSE OUTLINE

First aid is best learned by doing. You will use this book during this course to practice the steps for many of the emergencies listed in each section. In addition, you will learn how to assess an emergency, how to perform primary and secondary surveys, and how to properly move or transport a victim.

LEARNING GOALS

In this chapter you will learn about:

- Universal precautions
- The legal considerations of providing first aid
- The definition of first aid

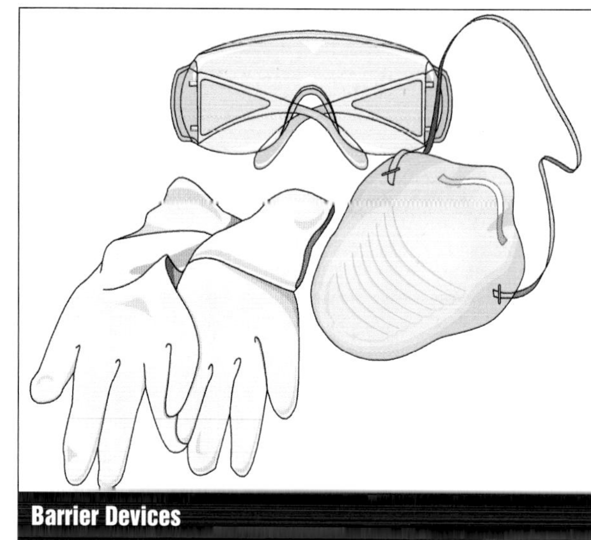

Barrier Devices

UNIVERSAL PRECAUTIONS

In 1987 the Centers for Disease Control and Prevention (CDC) in America first issued guidelines (called *Universal Precautions*) that everyone should follow when giving first aid. Universal Precautions means that you should consider blood and body fluids potentially infectious and you should take safety measures to protect yourself from them. These measures include:

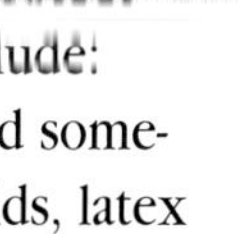

- Placing a barrier between you and someone else's body fluids. Face shields, latex gloves, and a pocket breathing mask are all examples of barrier devices.
- Covering any open sores, cuts, or scrapes you might have on your hands or exposed skin.
- Minimizing splashing body fluids.
- Handling any sharp objects with care.
- Not handling any food or drinks when providing first aid.
- Cleaning and disinfecting any area where body fluids have been spilled.
- Washing your hands and any exposed areas thoroughly, immediately after you have provided first aid or cleaned up a spill.

There has never been a documented case of anyone contracting a disease from using training aids and manikins during a first aid or CPR course. This is according to the CDC.

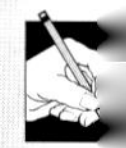

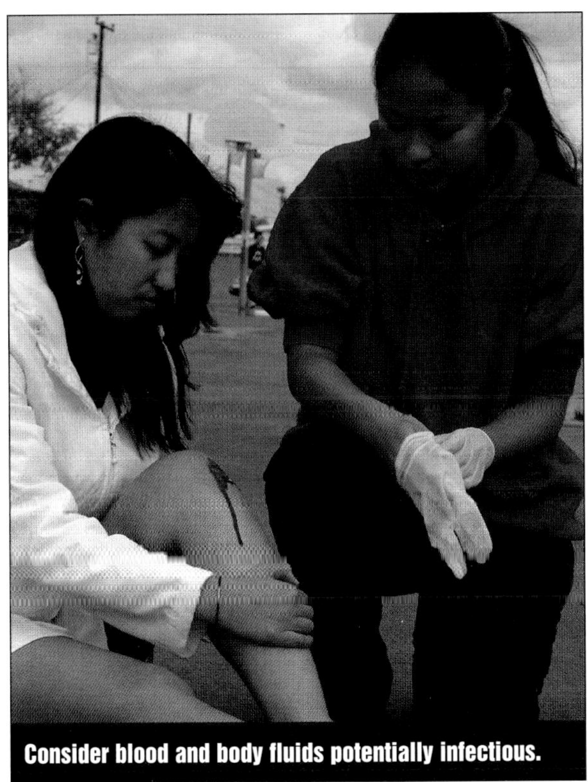
Consider blood and body fluids potentially infectious.

NAUI and your instructor follow the CDC's Guidelines for decontaminating and cleaning the manikins and training aids used during the First Aid course. As long as you follow instructions for decontamination during the course, your risk of contracting any kind of disease is extremely low. Always be sure to wash your hands before and after participating in any class activities. Also, do not eat, drink, or chew gum during class.

You should ask for a separate training manikin if any of the following situations apply to you:

- You have a cold or sore throat.
- You have open sores around your mouth or on your hands.
- You have a compromised immune system or condition that makes you unusually prone to getting an infection.
- You know you have a chronic infection such as AIDS, Hepatitis B, or Hepatitis C.
- You have tested positive for HIV antibodies.

You will not be asked to provide an explanation if you ask for a separate training manikin.

If you have any medical condition or disability that will prohibit you from participating in any of the physical skill sessions, please let your instructor know. They will make reasonable accommodations to enable you to participate.

LEGAL CONSIDERATIONS

You need to be aware of some basic legal considerations concerning first aid. It is highly unusual for a lawsuit to be brought against some one who provided care at an emergency scene.

Duty to Act

Some people have a duty to act in an emergency. These are *professional rescuers* on duty, such as licensed or certified professionals (including scuba instructors and dive leaders), public safety officers (firefighters and police), and medically trained personnel.

Good Samaritan Laws

Many jurisdictions have instituted Good Samaritan laws to protect people from liability as long as they:

- Act in a careful and sensible manner.
- Only provide care consistent with their training.
- Continue providing care until advanced medical help arrives and takes over.
- Do not accept anything in return for their services.

These laws vary from jurisdiction to jurisdiction. You can check with a legal service or your local library to find out the specific laws in your location. See "Example of a Good Samaritan Law."

Consent

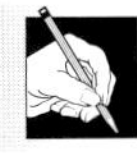

Before you can provide care for a *conscious* victim, you must have their consent. To obtain their consent:

- Tell them your name.

Florida Good Samaritan Law

768.13

Good Samaritan Act; immunity from civil liability.—

(1) This act shall be known and cited as the "Good Samaritan Act."

(2)(a) Any person, including those licensed to practice medicine, who gratuitously and in good faith renders emergency care or treatment either in direct response to emergency situations related to and arising out of a public health emergency declared pursuant to s. 381.00315, a state of emergency which has been declared pursuant to s. 252.36, or at the scene of an emergency outside of a hospital, doctor's office, or other place having proper medical equipment, without objection of the injured victim or victims thereof, shall not be held liable for any civil damages as a result of such care or treatment or as a result of any act or failure to act in providing or arranging further medical treatment where the person acts as an ordinary reasonably prudent person would have acted under the same or similar circumstances.

Example of a Good Samaritan Law

- Let them know that you have first aid training.
- Ask if you can help them.

If the victim is a minor, you must ask their parent or legal guardian for consent before you can help them.

If a victim is unconscious, is unable to respond, is confused, or is a minor with no adult supervision, they cannot give their consent for treatment. In these cases, the law assumes that the victim would have given consent if they were able to. This is called *implied consent*.

DEFINITION OF FIRST AID

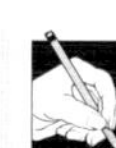

In the dictionary, *first aid* is emergency care given before regular medical aid can be obtained while a *rescue* is the removal from danger or the potential for further harm before first aid can begin.

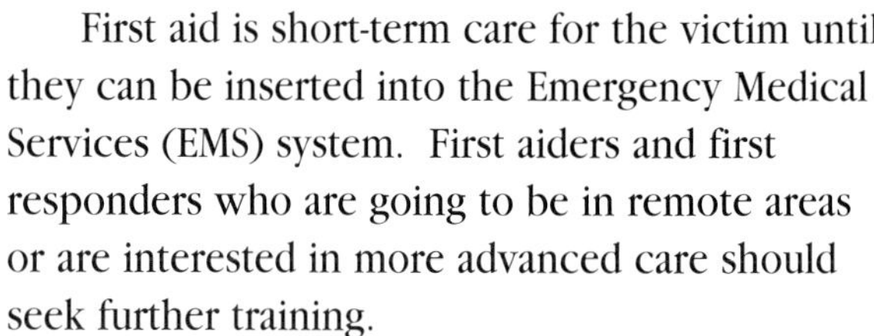

First aid is short-term care for the victim until they can be inserted into the Emergency Medical Services (EMS) system. First aiders and first responders who are going to be in remote areas or are interested in more advanced care should seek further training.

A rescue is the removal of a victim from danger or further harm. Sometimes, a rescue must be performed before first aid can be administered. During this course, you will learn some simple rescue principles along with the first aid for many different emergencies.

REVIEW QUESTIONS

1. Universal Precautions means that you should consider blood and body fluids __________ ______________.

2. There has never been a documented case of anyone contracting a disease from using _______________ and _____________during a first aid or CPR course.

3. Before you can provide care for a conscious victim, you must have their _____________ .

4. First aid is emergency care given ____ .

CHAPTER 2

Blood-Borne Pathogens

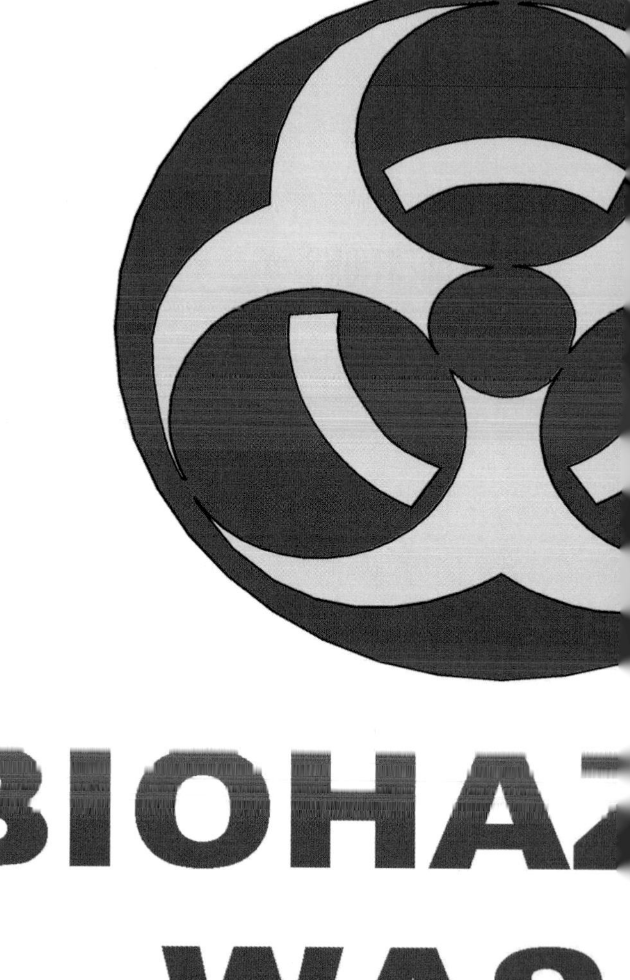

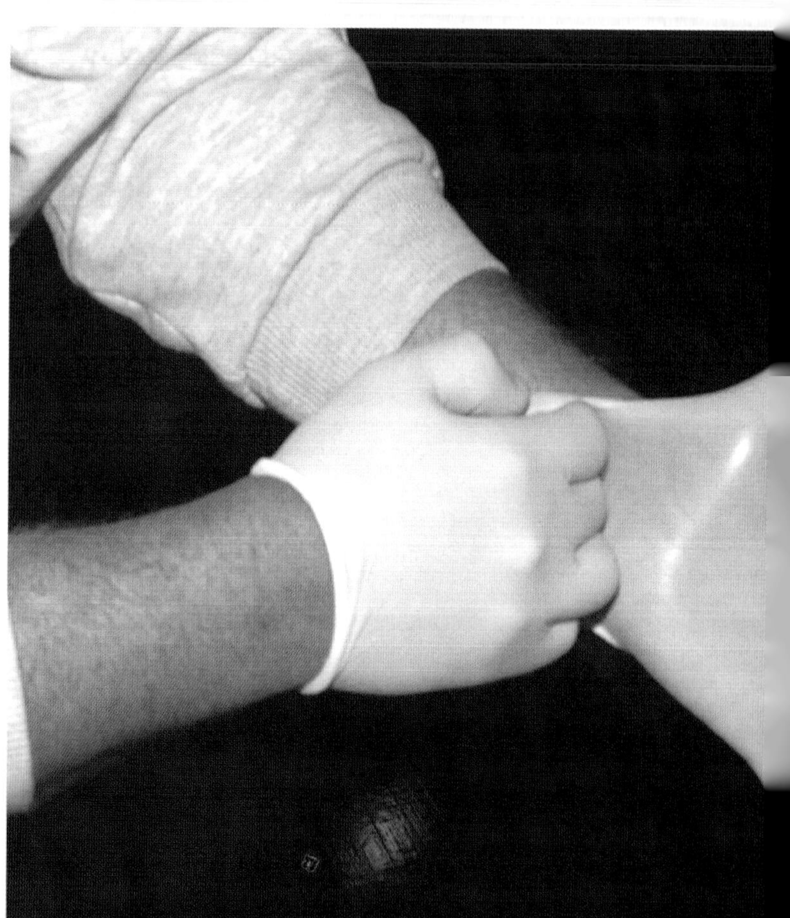

ARD

E

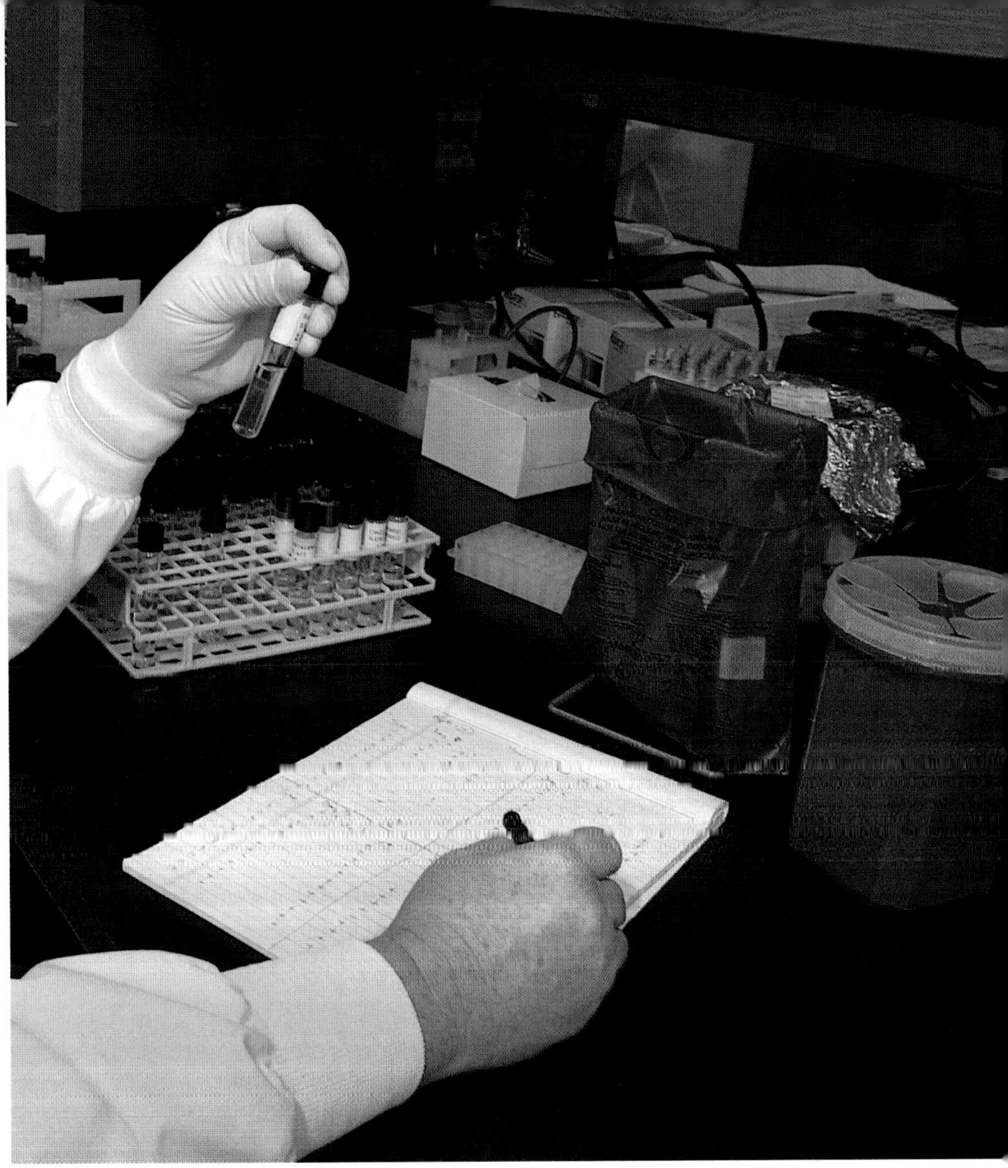

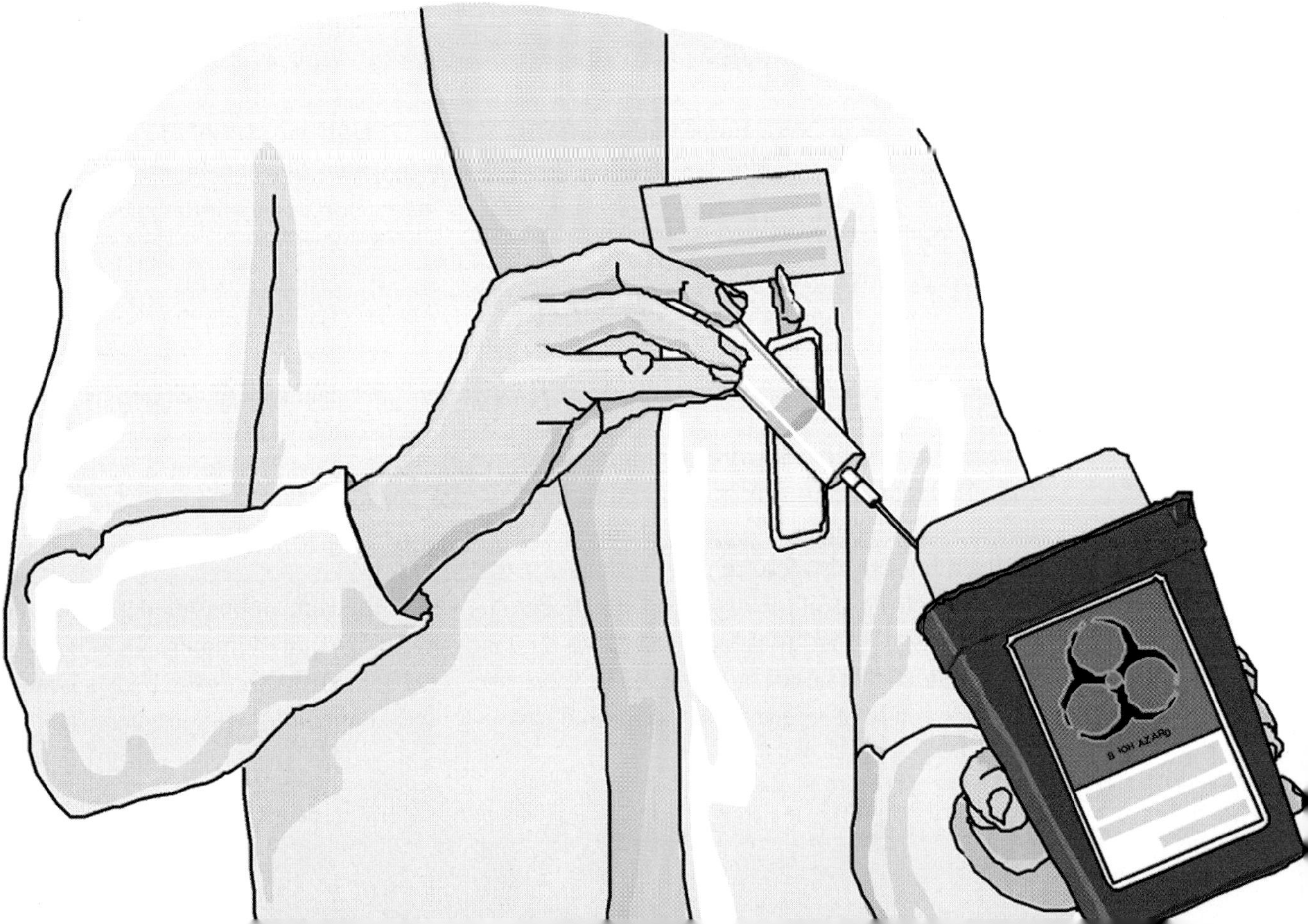

This chapter will make you aware of the different diseases that can be passed from one person to another through the blood or bodily fluids and how to reduce your risk of infection.

LEARNING GOALS

In this chapter you will learn about:

- Three types of blood-borne pathogens
- Modes of transmission for each pathogen
- Actions to take in the event of an exposure
- Labeling standards for biohazards

RELATED LEGISLATION AND LEGAL ISSUES

The United States Department of Labor Occupational Safety and Health Administration (OSHA) has a specific regulation for blood-borne pathogens. It is standard number 29 CFR 1910.1030. This standard was written to protect health-care workers who might come in contact with potentially infectious materials. For those interested in reviewing the law, a copy can be viewed via the internet at www.osha.gov.

BLOOD-BORNE PATHOGENS

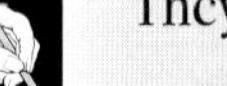

There are three blood-borne pathogens that are of primary concern to health-care workers. They are:

- Hepatitis B (HBV)
- Hepatitis C (HCV)
- Human Immunodeficiency Virus (HIV)

Hepatitis B

Hepatitis B (HBV) is a virus that infects the liver. Hepatitis B is usually transmitted through blood-to-blood contact. It causes inflammation of the liver, but can also lead to more serious diseases such as cirrhosis of the liver or liver cancer.

There is a vaccine available for Hepatitis B. It is recommended that health-care workers be vaccinated. Once you have received the vaccine and have developed immunity (by creating antibodies to the virus) you are at a very low risk for infection.

The signs and symptoms of a Hepatitis B infection can take from one to eight months to become noticeable after exposure to the virus. The signs and symptoms include:

- Fatigue
- Stomach pain
- Loss of appetite
- Nausea
- Jaundice (a distinct yellowing of the eyes and skin)
- Darkened urine

Hepatitis C

Hepatitis C (HCV) is also a virus that infects the liver. Hepatitis C can be transmitted through blood-to-blood contact. In 75% to 85% of infected people, it causes a chronic infection, and disease symptoms may not manifest for years after infection. In 70% of infected persons, it causes chronic liver disease. In one to five percent of infected people, it causes death from liver failure. Hepatitis C is the leading indication for a liver transplant. There is no vaccine available for Hepatitis C.

Eighty percent of the people with Hepatitis C have no signs or symptoms. For those who do have signs and symptoms, they include:

- Fatigue
- Stomach pain
- Loss of appetite
- Nausea
- Jaundice (a distinct yellowing of the eyes and skin)
- Darkened urine

HIV

The Human Immunodeficiency Virus (HIV) causes Acquired Immune Deficiency Syndrome (AIDS). HIV attacks the body's immune system, weakening it to a point where the body can no longer fight off other diseases. AIDS is fatal. A person can be infected with HIV, but it can be many years before AIDS develops. Control of HIV infection and treatment for AIDS is improving, but there is no cure for the disease.

HIV can be transmitted through blood-to-blood contact. HIV is an extremely fragile virus and cannot survive for long outside of the human body. The chance of contracting HIV in a work place environment is only about 0.4%. The signs and symptoms of an HIV infection include:

- Weakness
- Fever
- Sore throat
- Nausea
- Headaches
- Diarrhea
- White coating on the tongue
- Weight loss
- Swollen lymph glands

AIDS occurs in three stages. In the first stage, the person is infected with HIV. After the initial symptoms, the person might show only a few of the symptoms of illness for many years. In the second stage the person might have swollen lymph glands, and start to have problems fighting off other diseases. In the third stage, the person's body becomes completely unable to fight off other diseases and infections.

MODES OF TRANSMISSION

HBV, HCV, and HIV are all transmitted through contact with infected human blood or bodily fluids that enters your body through an open sore, cut, abrasion, acne, or any type of damaged or broken skin, or sexual transmission. Also, if the infected blood comes in contact with the mucus membranes in your eyes, nose, or mouth, it can transmit the virus to you. Other potentially infected body fluids are:

- Saliva
- Semen
- Vaginal secretions
- Cerebrospinal fluid
- Pleural fluid
- Peritoneal fluid
- Amniotic fluid

HBV, HCV, and HIV are most commonly transmitted through:

- Sexual contact (rare for HCV)
- Sharing hypodermic needles
- The placenta from a mother to a fetus
- Accidental puncture from a contaminated needle, broken glass, or other sharps
- Contact between broken skin or mucus membranes and contaminated body fluids

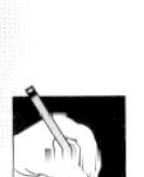

RISK ASSESSMENT

The risk of becoming infected by a blood-borne pathogen is fairly low. However, because of the seriousness of each disease, you must be careful not to come in contact with any contaminated body fluids. The risk for each blood-borne pathogen is as follows:

- HBV. The risk from a single exposure of HBV-infected blood to broken skin is from 6% to 30%. If a person has received Hepatitis B vaccine and has developed immunity to the virus, there is only a slight risk of infection.
- HCV. The risk from a single exposure of HCV-infected blood to broken skin is approximately 1.8%.
- HIV. The risk from a single exposure of HIV-infected blood to broken skin is approximately 0.3%. The risk from a single exposure of HIV-infected blood to the eye, nose, or mouth is 0.1%.

RISK MANAGEMENT

You can reduce your risk of becoming infected with a blood-borne pathogen by following universal precautions described in Chapter 1.

Vaccines

You can greatly reduce the risk of becoming infected with Hepatitis B virus through vaccination. For HCV, HBV, and HIV, you must follow the previously listed universal precautions to help prevent infections with HCV, HBV, and HIV.

IMMEDIATE ACTIONS TO TAKE IN THE EVENT OF AN EXPOSURE

If you come in contact with possibly contaminated body fluids, use the following steps:

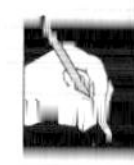

1. Perform one of the following procedures based on the type of contact:
   - Wash a puncture wound or any contaminated cuts with soap and water.
   - Flush splashes to the nose, mouth, or skin with fresh water.
   - Irrigate the eyes with fresh water, saline, or a sterile eye wash.
2. Report the exposure to your supervisor.
3. Fill out any necessary forms to document the exposure.
4. Seek the appropriate treatment (within 24 hours) for the pathogen to which you were exposed:
   - HBV. You can receive Hepatitis B immune globulin (HBIG) to prevent HBV infection. You can also receive the Hepatitis B vaccine (if you have not previously been vaccinated) at the same time.
   - HCV. There is no treatment after an exposure to HCV-infected body fluids. Receiving immune globulin or antiviral therapy is not recommended.
   - HIV. If your exposure poses a risk of infection, antiretroviral drugs will help reduce the chance of HIV transmission. However, if your exposure does not have a risk of HIV infection, the use of the antiretroviral drugs is not recommended due to the serious side effects.

FOLLOW-UP ACTIONS TO TAKE AFTER AN EXPOSURE

After an exposure, you should consider follow-up treatment, based on the pathogen to which you are exposed:

- HBV. Routine follow-up is not needed if you have received Hepatitis B immune globulin or have been vaccinated for Hepatitis B. You should be tested one to two months after receiving the Hepatitis B vaccine to see if you have developed immunity to Hepatitis B. If you develop signs or symptoms of Hepatitis B, you should see your healthcare provider.
- HCV. You should be tested for the HCV antibody and liver enzyme levels as soon as possible after the exposure and then again four to six months after the exposure. You can also be tested for presence of the HCV virus four to six weeks after the exposure. If you develop signs or symptoms of Hepatitis C, you should see your healthcare provider. Currently, multiple-drug treatments can reduce the risk of disease.
- HIV. You should be tested for the HIV antibody as soon as possible after the exposure and then periodically for the next six months after exposure. If you take the antiretroviral drugs, you should be tested for a complete blood count and kidney and liver function tests before starting the treatment and then again two weeks after starting the treatment. This will check for drug toxicity in your system. If you have any signs or symp-

toms of a sudden or severe flu-like illness, see your healthcare provider. These signs and symptoms might indicate HIV infection or a drug reaction. During the treatment period, it is best to follow the recommendations for preventing the transmission of blood-borne pathogens:

- Do not donate blood, semen, or organs.
- Do not have sexual intercourse, or use a condom consistently and correctly.
- Do not breast feed infants.

LABELING STANDARDS

Biohazard labels need to be affixed to the following items:

- Containers of regulated waste:
  - Liquid or semi-liquid blood or other potentially infectious materials
  - Contaminated items that might release blood or other potentially infectious materials if compressed
  - Items that are caked with dried blood or other potentially infectious materials and that might release these materials during handling.
  - Contaminated sharps containers
  - Pathological and microbiological wastes containing blood or other potentially infectious materials
- Refrigerators or freezers containing blood or other potentially infectious materials
- Containers used to store or ship blood or other potentially infectious materials

Biohazard labels are fluorescent orange, red, or orange-red. The bags used to dispose of blood or other potentially infectious materials are also red or orange-red and have the biohazard symbol prominently stamped on the bag. Regulated waste should be double-bagged in case the outer bag is punctured.

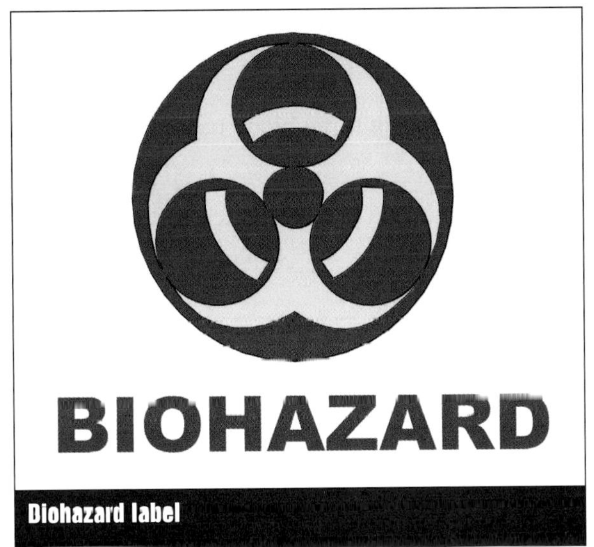

Biohazard label

INFORMATION RESOURCES

Three good resources of information about blood-borne pathogens are:

- The World Health Organization (WHO). Their internet site is www.who.int/en/.
- The United States Department of Labor Occupational Safety and Health Administration (OSHA). OSHA has developed the "Blood-Borne Pathogens Standard 1910.1030." Their internet site is www.osha.gov.
- The United States Department of Health and Human Services Centers for Disease Control and Prevention (CDC). Their internet site is www.cdc.gov.

REVIEW QUESTIONS

1. There are three blood-borne pathogens; they are ____________________(______) ____________________(______), ____________________(______).
2. HBV, HCV, and HIV are most commonly transmitted through:
   - ____________contact (rare for HCV).
   - Sharing __________________ ____________________.
   - ______________________________ from a mother to a fetus.
   - Accidental _______________ from a contaminated _________, _________, or other ________________.
   - Contact between ________________ or ________________ and contaminated body fluids.
3. If you come in contact with possibly contaminated body fluids, use the following steps: Perform one of the following procedures based on the type of contact:
   - Wash a puncture wound or any contaminated cuts with ___________ _____________.
   - Flush splashes to the ______, _______, or _______ with ______ ____.
   - Irrigate the ______ with ______ _______, _______, or a _________ _________ _______.
4. Biohazard labels are ____.

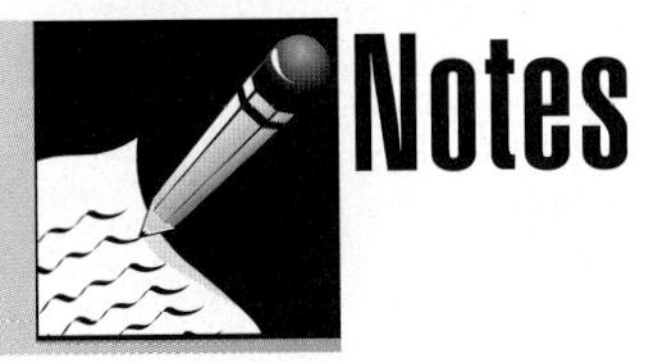

Notes

CHAPTER 3

Human Anatomy

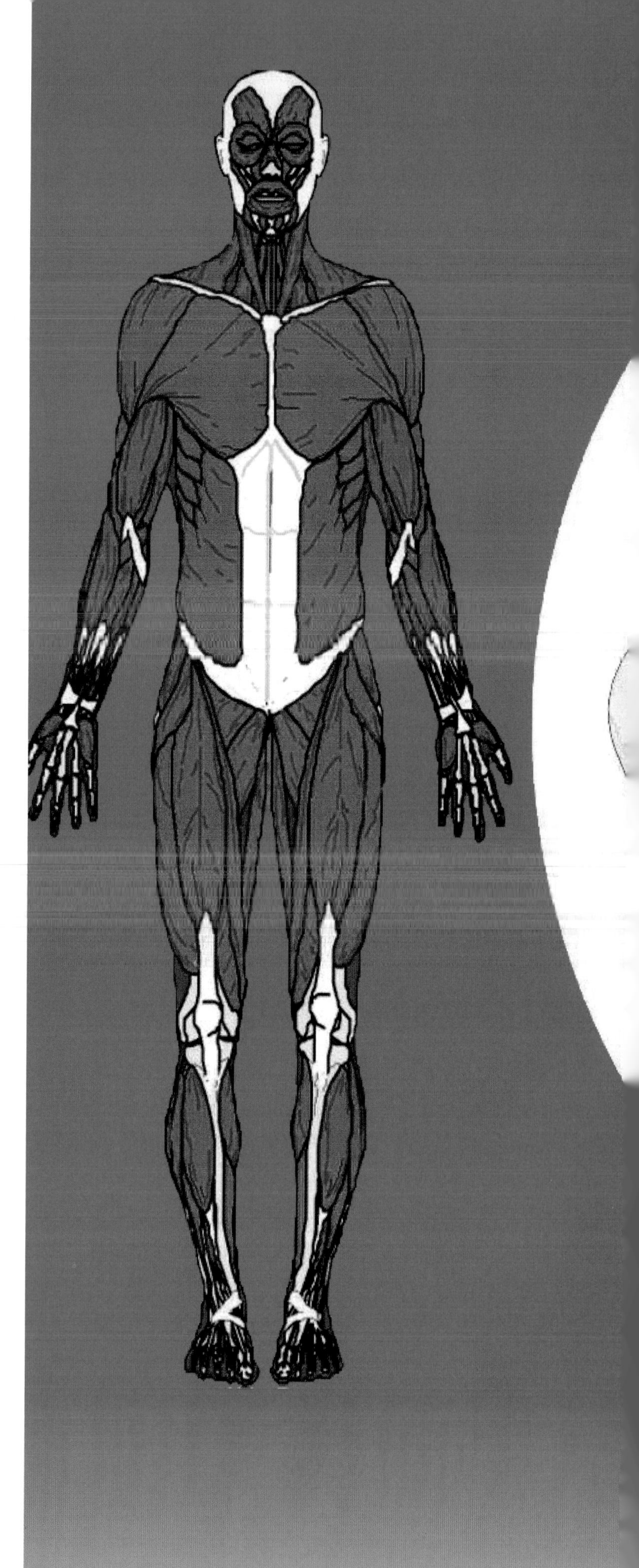

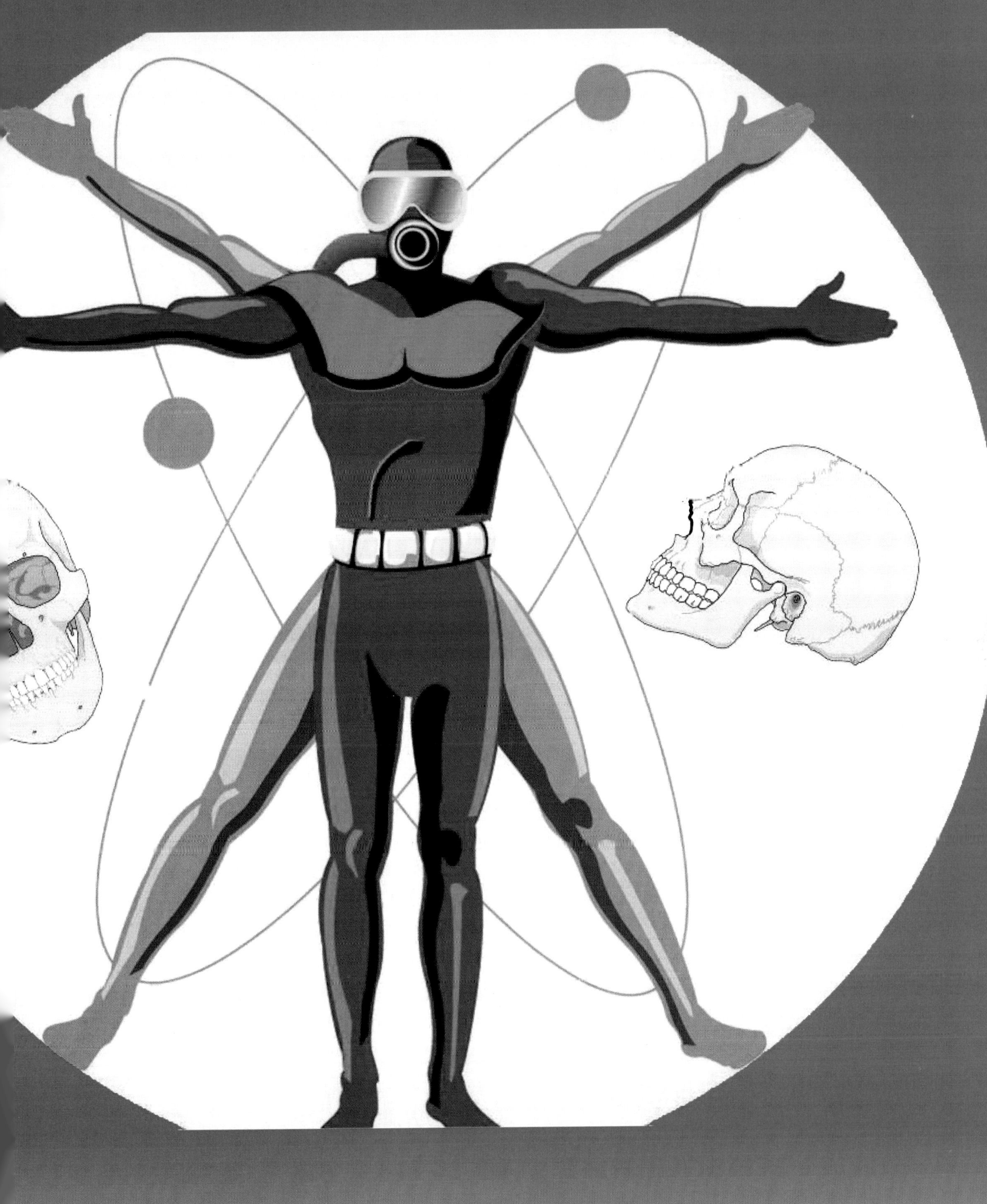

Effectively providing first aid to an injured person will require some rudimentary knowledge of human anatomy.

LEARNING GOALS

In this chapter you will learn about:

- Bodily systems
- Pulse points
- Taking pulses
- Breathing mechanics
- Parts of the body

Just as an auto mechanic must know the parts and systems of the vehicle and how they interact in order to repair it, a basic knowledge of the workings of the human body is helpful when diagnosing an injury or illness and providing the first aid that is required.

SYSTEMS

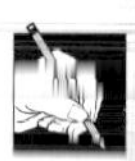

The human body is composed of 10 major systems, 5 of which may be involved in the majority of first aid situations.

- Cardiovascular
- Respiratory
- Musculoskeletal
- Nervous
- Integumentary (Skin)

Others, while important to human function are not normally considered during first aid:

- Digestive
- Urinary
- Endocrine
- Lymphatic
- Reproductive

CARDIOVASCULAR SYSTEM

The cardiovascular (circulatory) system controls the circulation of the blood and the products that it carries throughout the body. It includes the blood, heart, and blood vessels.

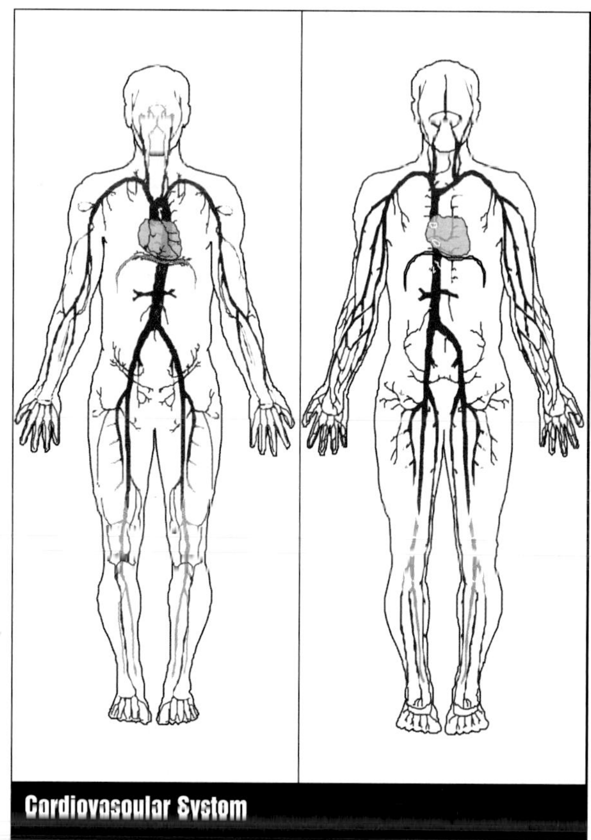

Cardiovascular System

Blood

Blood is the medium that transports oxygen from the respiratory system to the body's cells. The blood also carries other chemicals, proteins, and hormones that are essential to the function of the human body. Waste products, including carbon dioxide, which is transported to the lungs for expulsion, are carried away from the cells by the blood.

The average adult body contains approximately 5 liters (a little more than 5 quarts) of blood. The volume of blood in the body is circulated completely throughout the body approximately 1,000 times a day or once every 1 to 1.5 minutes.

Heart

The heart is a 4-chamber pump that moves the blood through the blood vessels. The heart is divided by a septum into right and left sides.

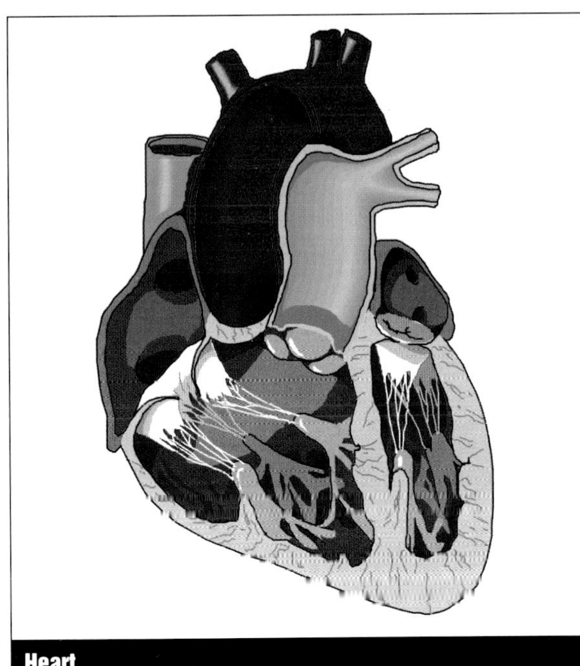

Heart

The left side receives oxygenated blood from the lungs and sends it to the body. The right side receives deoxygenated blood from the body and sends it to the lungs. Each side is further divided into 2 halves. The top half is known as the atrium and the bottom half, the ventricle. These halves work in tandem with each other to move the blood through the heart. The atrium receives the blood coming from the body or the lungs. When the atrium contracts, sending blood to the ventricle, the ventricle below expands to receive the blood. Then the ventricle contracts to push the blood out of the heart, and the atrium expands to bring blood in. A one-way valve prevents backflow from the ventricle to the atrium.

The average human heart beats between 50 and 95 times per minute. Each beat creates a pulse that can be palpated (felt) at several locations or "pulse points" throughout the body. When the heart contracts and pushes blood out, "blood pressure" is created against the walls of the arteries as the blood passes through them. Blood pressure is measured in millimeters of mercury (mmHg) with the normal or average blood pressure being about

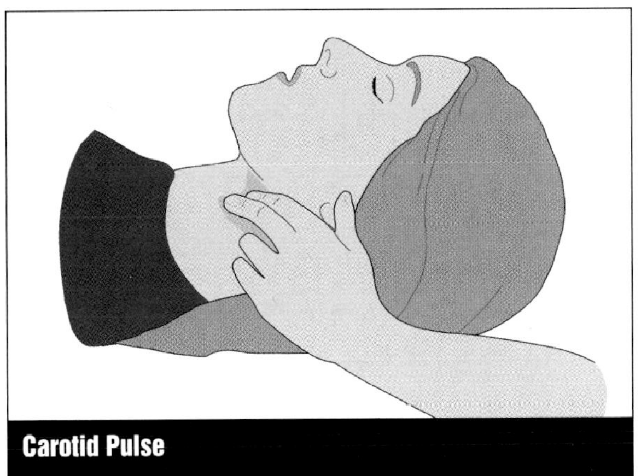

Carotid Pulse

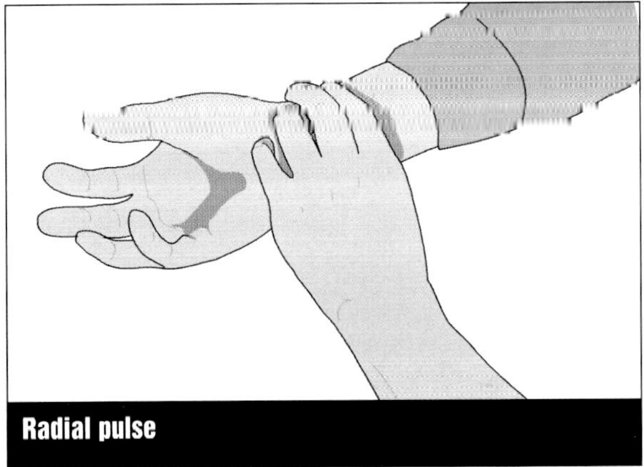

Radial pulse

120/80 mmHg. Systole is the contraction of the heart muscle. The pressure of the blood measured at that time is known as systolic pressure. This is the first or higher number noted when reading blood pressure. Diastole is the term for the relaxation of the heart. The blood pressure at that time is known as diastolic blood pressure measurement and is the lower number on a blood pressure.

Pulse Points

It is important that the first aid provider be able to locate the 8 most common pulse points used during first aid operations and the arteries that they indicate; 2 carotid, 2 radial, 2 brachial, and 2 femoral.

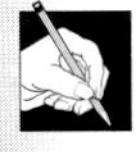

The carotid and radial pulses are most commonly used to determine presence and quality of circulation. The carotid artery (pulse) can be

found on either side of the neck and is located in the groove just to the side and behind the larynx (windpipe). The radial artery (pulse) is located on the inner surface of the wrist next to the tendon at the base of the thumb.

While brachial and femoral pulse points might also determine presence of circulation, these are more often used to control bleeding in the arms and legs, respectively. The brachial artery can be found inside the arm between the bicep and triceps muscles and about 5 centimeters (2 inches) above the inside of the elbow, where the brachial artery crosses over the humerus (upper arm bone). The femoral artery can be felt on the upper, inner thigh in the fold where it meets the groin.

Taking Pulses

A slow heart beat, cold, and other factors can make detecting a pulse difficult. The first aid provider should always take at least 10 seconds when checking for the presence of circulation.

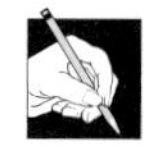

Radial pulse: Using the 2nd and 3rd finger preferably, place them on the inside in the groove that lies just at the base of the arm on the inside where it joins the wrist. Move the fingers up and down or side to side until the pulse is felt. Be careful to not use the thumb to take a pulse. It can sometimes exhibit its own pulse, and you may mistake your own for that of the victim.

Carotid pulse: Using the same 2 fingers, place them on the larynx (windpipe) and then slide them towards the side until they enter a groove between the windpipe and the muscle. The carotid pulse can be palpated in that groove. Since the carotid artery supplies blood to the brain, do not press hard or long enough to cut off the blood supply through the artery. NEVER CHECK BOTH RIGHT AND LEFT SIDES AT THE SAME TIME. If you do so, you might cause the body to react to the bilateral pressure by dropping an already low blood pressure dangerously low.

Brachial pulse: Using the 2nd, 3rd and 4th fingers press on the inside of the arm between the bicep and triceps muscles. The brachial pulse can be felt in that groove. If using as a pulse point, press just hard enough to detect the pulse. If controlling bleeding, press hard enough to compress the vessel against the humerus and slow or stop the major flow of blood to the arm.

Femoral pulse: The femoral artery lies deep in the leg and is the most difficult to feel or control. For this reason, the femoral artery is seldom used to detect a pulse. (Finding the pulse to a leg is normally done using one of two pulse points in the foot.) However, the femoral artery may be used to control bleeding in the legs. To control bleeding using the femoral pressure point, the victim should be lying on their back with the first aid provider at their feet. Push hard with the heel of your hand up into the fold between the upper thigh and the groin. This will compress the femoral artery against the pelvis and slow or stop the major flow of blood to the leg.

Blood Vessels and Circulation

There are 5 types of blood vessels in the cardiovascular system: arteries, arterioles, capillaries, venules, and veins. Arteries and arterioles carry blood away from the heart. Venules and veins carry blood toward the heart. Capillaries are the link between them.

Oxygenated blood travels from the lungs through the pulmonary vein to the left atrium and then into the left ventricle. The blood leaves the ventricle through the aorta (the body's largest artery) and continues on through other arteries to the various parts of the body. As the arteries travel away from the heart, they narrow and become arterioles, which eventually meet with the capillaries, the smallest blood vessels. The capillaries essentially serve all parts of the body and are the site at which the oxygen that is carried from the lungs and heart by the blood is exchanged for the carbon dioxide that has been produced by metabolism in the cells. After passing through the capillaries, the deoxygenated, high-carbon dioxide blood enters the venules and then passes via the veins to the right atrium and the right ventricle and exits the heart through the pulmonary artery. As previously described, the pulmonary artery narrows into arterioles and eventually meets the pulmonary capillaries surrounding the air sacs (alveoli) in the lungs. This is where the gas exchange takes place as the carbon dioxide diffuses from the blood into the lungs, and the oxygen passes from the lungs into the blood, where it bonds chemically to the hemoglobin in the red blood cells. After giving up carbon dioxide and picking up oxygen, the blood continues through venules and then veins until it again reaches the left atrium, where the process begins again.

First Aid Implications

The first aid provider may be called upon to locate and use pulse points to evaluate the presence and quality of circulation and to perform chest compressions if circulation is absent.

RESPIRATORY SYSTEM

The respiratory system carries inhaled, oxygen-rich air into the lungs, allows for the exchange of oxygen in the lungs for carbon dioxide in the blood and then expels the oxygen poor, carbon dioxide-rich air from the lungs.

Structures of the Respiratory System

The respiratory system is made up of the trachea, the bronchi, the bronchioles, the lungs (with their alveoli), and the diaphragm. Air enters the body through the mouth and nose and passes into the trachea, which divides into 2 bronchi (one for each lung) and then into the smaller bronchioles, which further subdivide into still smaller bronchioles. At the end of each bronchiole is a cluster of air sacs known as the alveoli. Pulmonary capillaries surround the alveoli and it is here where oxygen in the lungs will be exchanged for carbon dioxide in the blood.

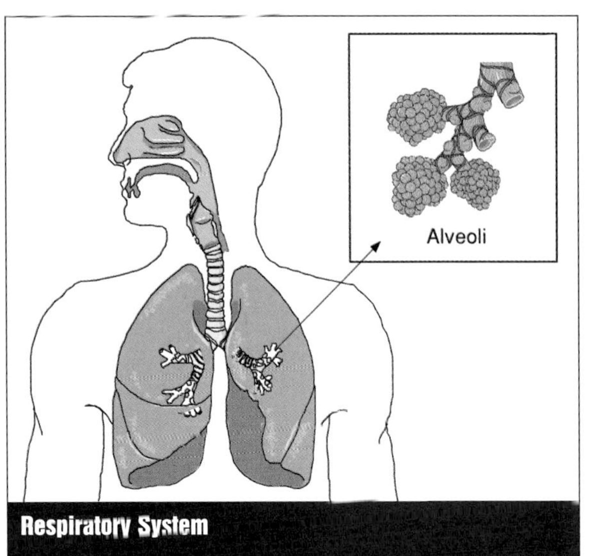

Respiratory System

Breathing Mechanics and Oxygen / Carbon Dioxide Exchange

The diaphragm is a flat, dome-shaped muscle that extends up into the thoracic (chest) cavity and forms the lower boundary of the thorax. When it contracts and pulls down, the thorax and lungs become larger, and the air pressure within the lungs decreases. This decreased pressure pulls air through the nose and mouth to flow into the trachea and eventually to the alveoli.

When the alveoli are inflated, they refill with air containing approximately 21% oxygen. The capillaries surrounding the alveoli contain blood that has come from the tissues and is low in oxygen (deoxygenated) and high in carbon dioxide. Gas exchange occurs as these gasses move from the area of higher concentration to one of lower.

When the diaphragm relaxes, it returns to its normal shape pushing up into the thorax, increasing the pressure around the lungs and forcing the air out of the alveoli through the bronchioles, bronchi, trachea, and eventually out through the mouth and nose.

When we exhale, we breathe out air that is lower in oxygen and higher in carbon dioxide. The air that we inhale is approximately 21% oxygen and has only a trace of carbon dioxide; the air

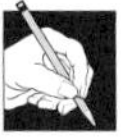

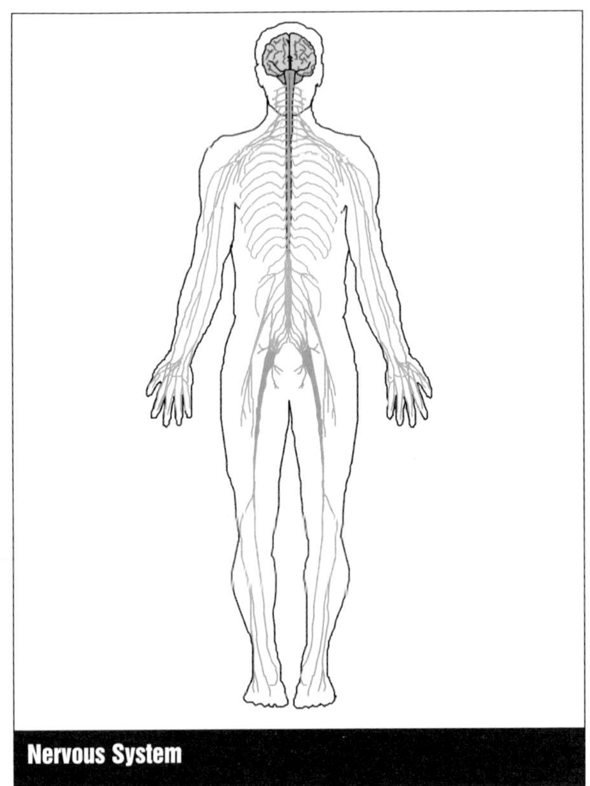

Nervous System

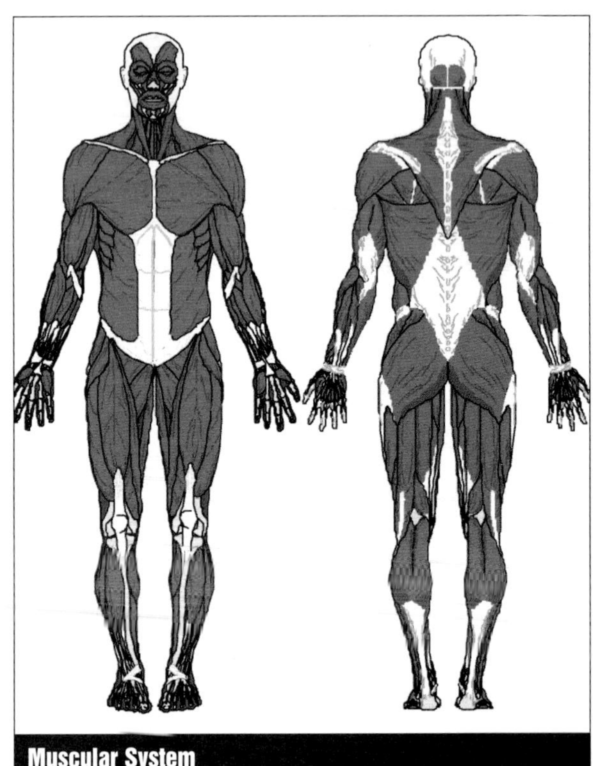

Muscular System

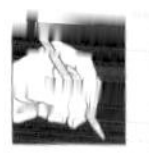

that we exhale is approximately 16% oxygen and 5% carbon dioxide.

This process repeats approximately 12 times per minute in the average adult human.

First Aid Implications

The first aid provider may need to assess the presence and quality of respiration and provide artificial respiration (rescue breathing) to the victim if inadequate or absent.

NERVOUS SYSTEM

The brain and spinal cord make up the central nervous system. The nerves that branch off the spinal cord comprise the peripheral nervous system. These together comprise the nervous system.

The brain is the organ that primarily controls the functions of the body. The spinal cord is made up of nerves that originate in the brain and travel down from the brain stem through the protection of the 33 bones of the spinal column. The peripheral nervous system is made up of 31 pairs of peripheral nerves. At each vertebra, a pair of peripheral nerves split and exit the spinal column and extend out to the various organs and tissues that they serve.

First Aid Implications

Injuries to the brain or spine can cause other systems to fail. The first aid provider will need to identify these injuries and offer support to those systems that are not functioning properly due to the nervous system injury.

MUSCULOSKELETAL SYSTEM

Muscles

Muscles are tissues that provide the body the ability to move. The more than 600 muscles in the body can be divided into 3 types; cardiac, skeletal, and smooth.

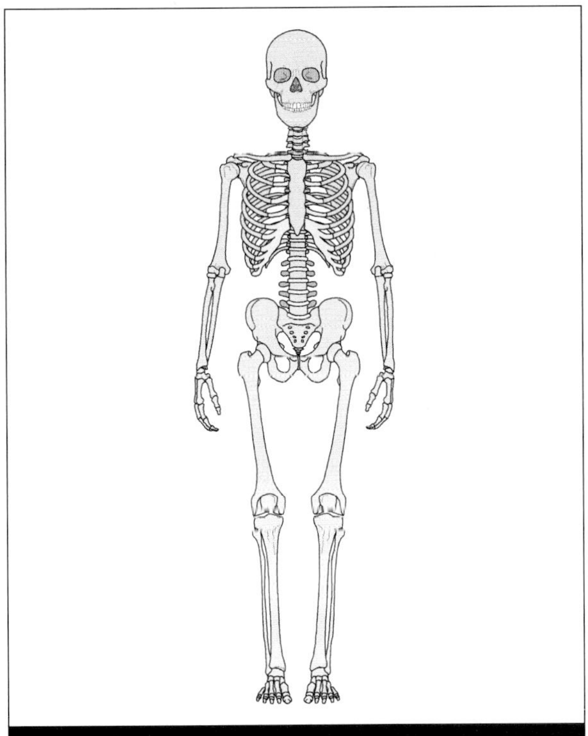
Skeletal System

The walls of the heart are made up of a specially modified muscle known as cardiac muscle. Unlike other muscles that often rest, the cardiac muscle must function constantly. It is, therefore, provided with a very rich blood supply and by way of the coronary arteries is the first organ to receive oxygenated blood after it leaves the heart.

Skeletal muscle attaches to the bones and makes up the majority of the body's muscle mass. Unlike the cardiac muscle, which operates independently of consciousness or thought, skeletal muscle is known as voluntary because it can be stimulated to contract or relax as one needs or desires.

Most involuntary actions, other than that which controls the heart, are controlled by the smooth muscles. Smooth muscle is found in the internal organs, major blood vessels, and other systems that respond to stimuli such as heat or the need to eliminate waste.

The diaphragm is another specialized muscle having characteristics of both the voluntary skeletal muscle and the involuntary smooth muscle. While the muscle operates mostly involuntarily, it can voluntarily be controlled, for example when one holds their breath.

Skeleton

206 bones make up the human body. The skeleton gives the body shape, allows for movement, protects the internal organs, serves as a source of calcium and other body chemicals, and produces red blood cells. The skeletal divisions and the bones they contain are:

- Skull - 22
  - 8 cranial bones
  - 14 facial bones
- Ears and Throat - 7
  - 3 in each ear
  - 1 floating (hyoid) in the throat under the tongue

Note: The hyoid is the only bone in the body that does not articulate with (touch) another bone.

- Spinal Column - 24
  - 7 cervical (neck) vertebrae
  - 12 thoracic (chest) vertebrae
  - 5 lumbar (lower back) vertebrae
- Rib Cage - 25
  - 12 pairs of ribs
  - 1 sternum
- Shoulder Girdle - 4
  - 2 clavicles
  - 2 scapulae
- Arms - 6
  - 2 humeri (singular: humerus)
  - 2 radii (singular: radius)
  - 2 ulnas
- Hands - 54
  - 27 each
- Pelvic Girdle - 4
  - 2 pelvic bones
  - 1 sacrum (5 fused into 1)
  - 1 coccyx
- Legs - 8
  - 2 femurs
  - 2 patellas (kneecap)

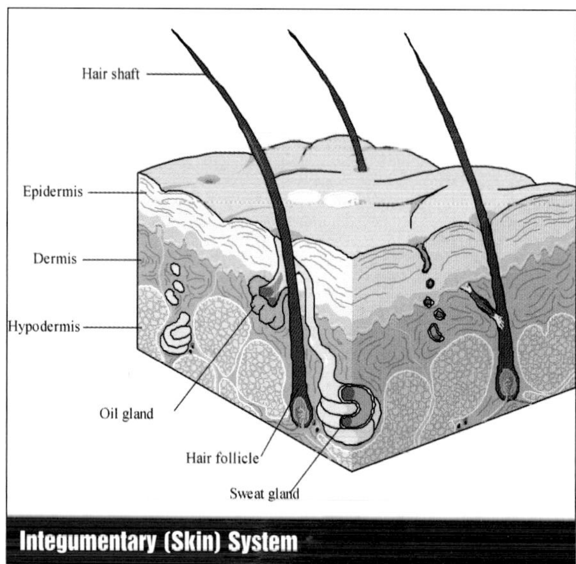

Integumentary (Skin) System

- 2 tibias
- 2 fibulas

• Feet - 52
- 26 each

First Aid Implications

Sprains and strains to muscles and broken and fractured bones are common first aid injuries. Knowledge of the skeletal system will assist the first aid provider during the patient assessment.

INTEGUMENTARY (SKIN) SYSTEM

The largest organ in the body is the skin. This organ protects the body, regulates its temperature, and transmits information to the brain from the environment.

The skin has 2 parts, the epidermis, which is actually made up of several layers, and the dermis (lower layer) that contains several specialized skin structures such as sweat glands and hair follicles.

First Aid Implications

Cuts, bruises and burns are all skin injuries that may require action by the first aid provider.

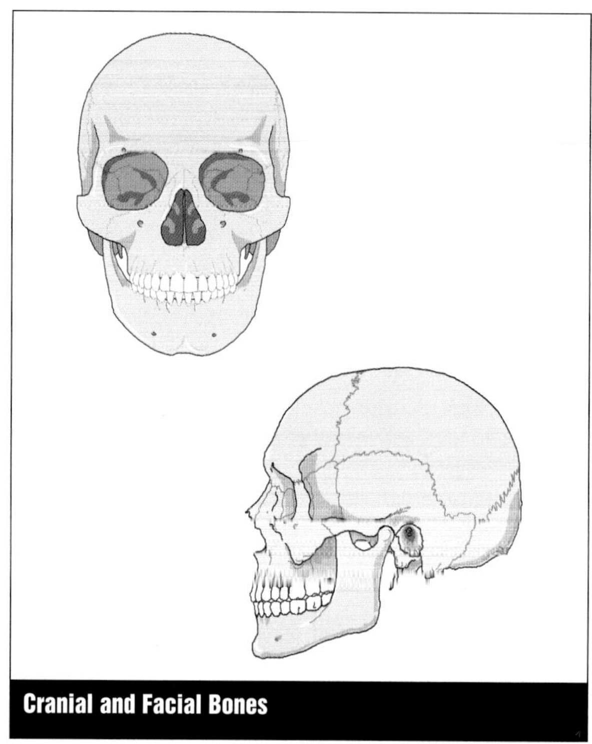
Cranial and Facial Bones

PARTS OF THE BODY

The human body can also be viewed in sections or parts, each of which may contain parts or elements of some or all of the systems described above. A working knowledge of these parts and their topography is important to the first aid provider during the primary and secondary (head-to-toe) victim assessment. The major divisions of the body are:

- Head
- Neck
- Upper Extremities
- Thorax
- Abdomen
- Pelvis
- Lower Extremities

Head

The head is divided into 2 parts, the cranium and the face, separated by an imaginary horizontal line passing across the top of the eyes and ears.

The cranium, the area above the line, contains the brain. The scalp is the skin covering the cranium. The face, the area below the line, contains the eyes, ears, nose, and mouth.

First Aid Implications

Head injuries may involve attention to nervous system injury, fractures to the skull, or cuts to the scalp.

Neck

The neck consists of several parts. The neck supports the head on the first 7 vertebrae of the spine, the cervical vertebrae. The spinal cord from the brain travels through and is protected by these cervical vertebrae.

The neck also contains the upper portions of the esophagus and trachea (windpipe) as well as the carotid arteries and jugular veins.

First Aid Implications

Neck injuries can be very severe if there is damage to the cervical spine and, more importantly, the spinal cord that it protects. Proper attention and care must be taken when addressing neck injuries to prevent further injury.

Upper Extremities

The upper extremities are composed of the clavicle and scapula (shoulder girdle), upper arm, elbow, lower arm, wrist and the hand and fingers.

The upper arm (humerus) extends from the shoulder to the elbow. The radius and ulna continue to the wrist, which joins the hand and the 27 bones that it contains.

First Aid Implications

Injuries to the upper extremities are mostly musculoskeletal including dislocation, breaks, and fractures. Burns, cuts, and bruises to the skin covering those structures are also common.

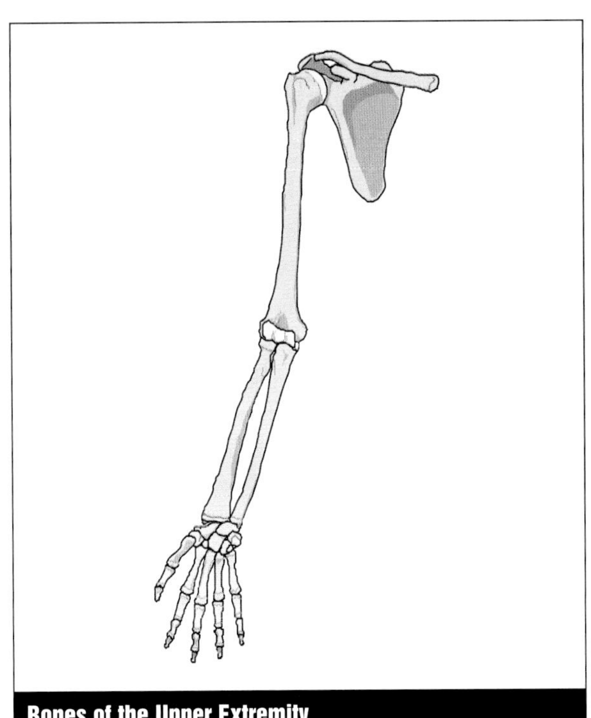

Bones of the Upper Extremity

Thorax

The thorax contains the heart and the major vessels that take blood from and to the heart (aorta and two venae cavae). It also contains the lungs and the lower portions of the trachea and esophagus.

These organs and vessels are bounded and protected by the 12 thoracic vertebrae in the back and the 12 pair of ribs that connect to those vertebrae and circle around to the front. The first 7 ribs connect to the sternum (breastbone). The remaining 5 do not connect directly to the sternum in the front and are referred to as "floating."

The sternum is made up of 3 parts; the upper quarter (manubrium), the lower three-quarters (body), and a cartilaginous tip at the bottom known as the xiphoid process. During CPR, proper chest compressions will be applied to the body of the sternum between the nipples and thereby avoid pushing the xiphoid process downward into the underlying organs.

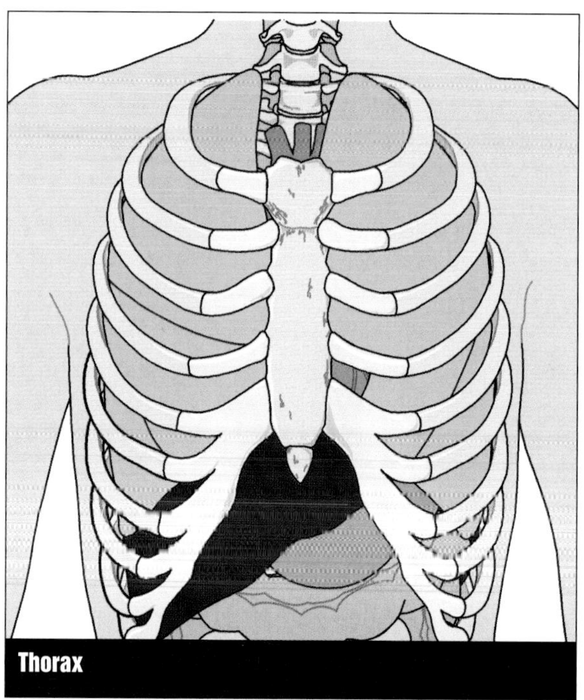
Thorax

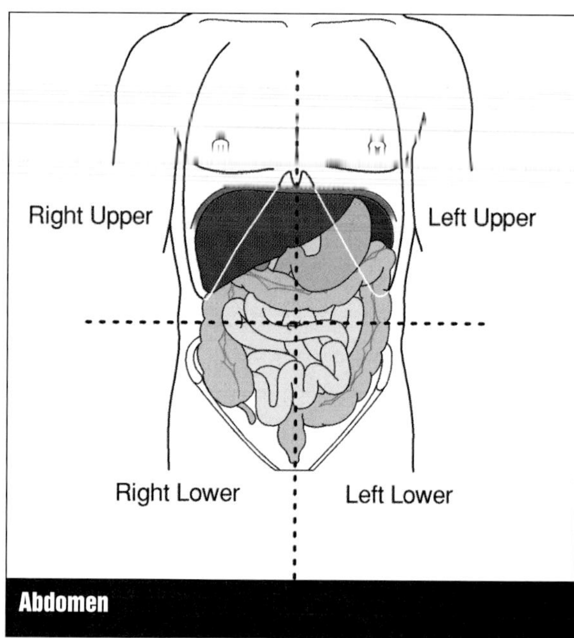

Abdomen

The diaphragm, a large flat dome-shaped muscle that assists in breathing, separates the thorax from the abdomen.

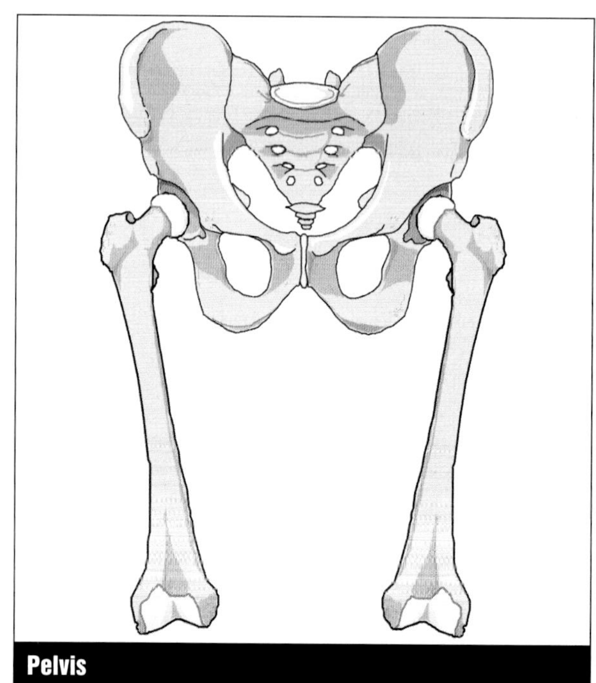
Pelvis

First Aid Implications

Injuries to the thorax can include or lead to broken ribs, damage to the heart and lungs, and respiratory and cardiac arrest. Life-threatening injuries will often include some injury to the thorax and the organs that it contains and protects.

Abdomen

The abdomen contains the major organs of digestion and excretion and is described by referring to 4 quadrants: right upper, left upper, right lower and left lower. Right and left refer to the victim's right and left.

The right upper quadrant contains the gall bladder and the largest portion of the liver. The left upper quadrant contains the stomach and spleen. The small intestine and large intestine (colon) lie in all 4 quadrants.

First Aid Implications

Injury to the abdomen can cause damage to its internal components and often lead to internal

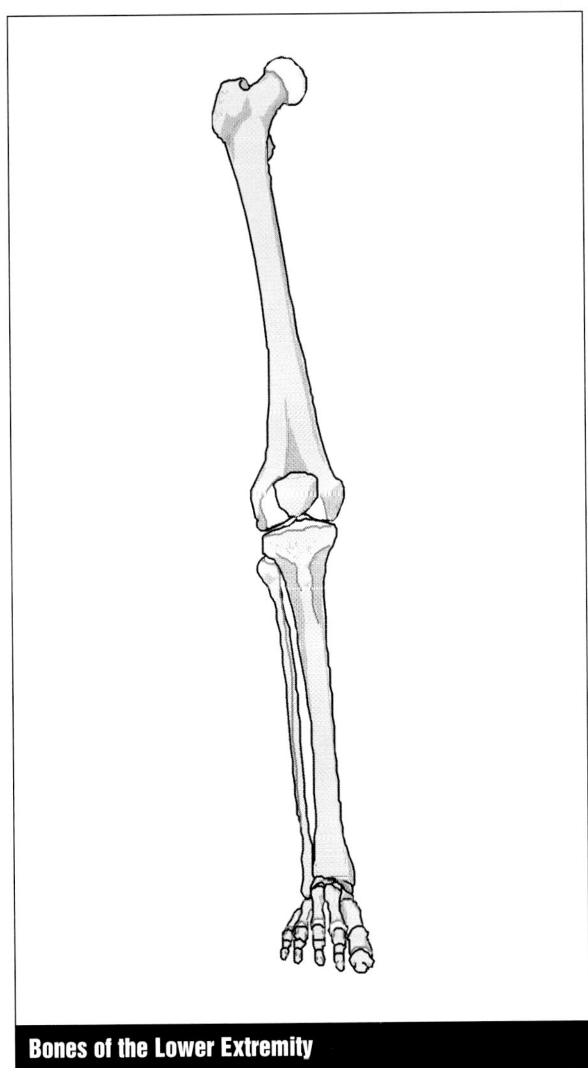

Bones of the Lower Extremity

bleeding that is difficult for the first aid provider to address. It will be important to quickly identify these types of injuries and seek appropriate medical attention.

Pelvis

The pelvis is a bony ring consisting of 4 bones (2 pelvic bones, the sacrum and the coccyx) and supports the upper part of the body on top of the lower extremities.

First Aid Implications

Injuries to the pelvis are similar to those of the upper extremities.

Lower Extremities

The lower extremities are comprised of the thigh, upper leg, knee, lower leg, ankle, and foot. The hip is the joint between the pelvic girdle and thigh. The primary structure of the upper leg is the femur, which runs from the hip to the knee, the joint between the thigh and lower leg. The tibia and fibula extend from the knee to the ankle, the joint between the lower leg and foot. The foot is made up of 26 bones.

First Aid Implications

Injuries to the lower extremities are similar to those of the upper extremities.

REVIEW QUESTIONS

1. The human body is composed of ________________, ___ of which may be involved in the majority of first aid situations.
2. The average adult body contains approximately ________ (________________) of blood.
3. The 8 most common pulse points used during first aid operations and the arteries that they indicate are: ____ ____.
4. The first aid provider should always take at least ______________ when checking for the presence of circulation.
5. The air that we inhale is approximately __________ and has only a trace of ____________; the air that we exhale is approximately __________ and ________________.
6. The major divisions of the body are: ____ ____

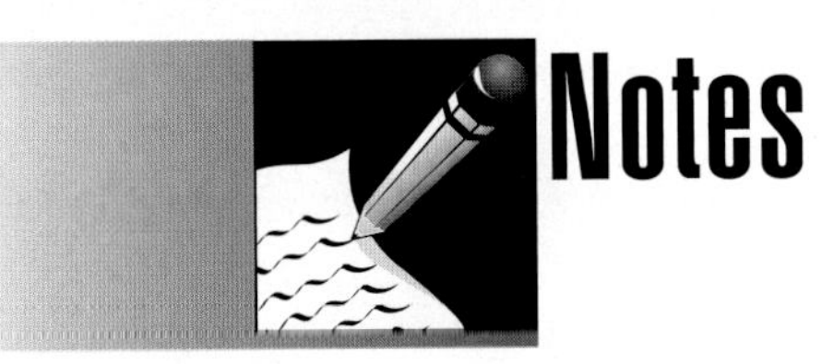

Notes

CHAPTER 4

Emergency Response and Victim Assessment

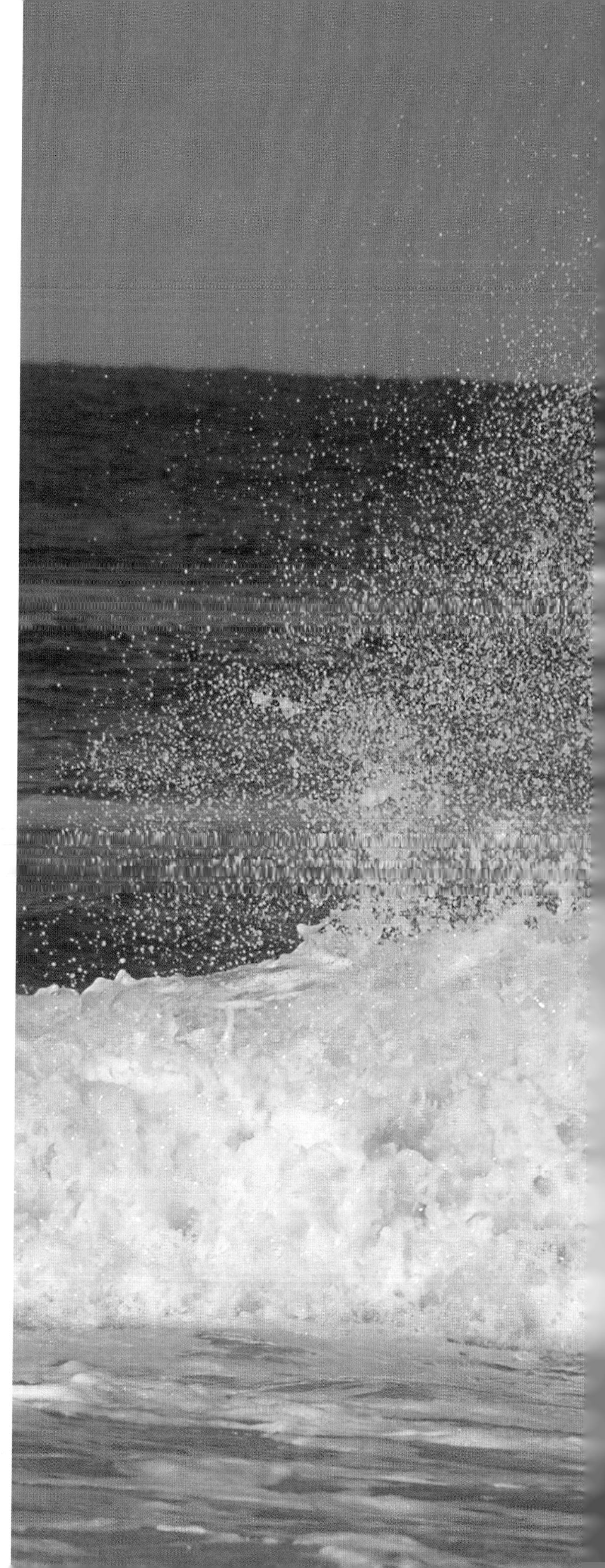

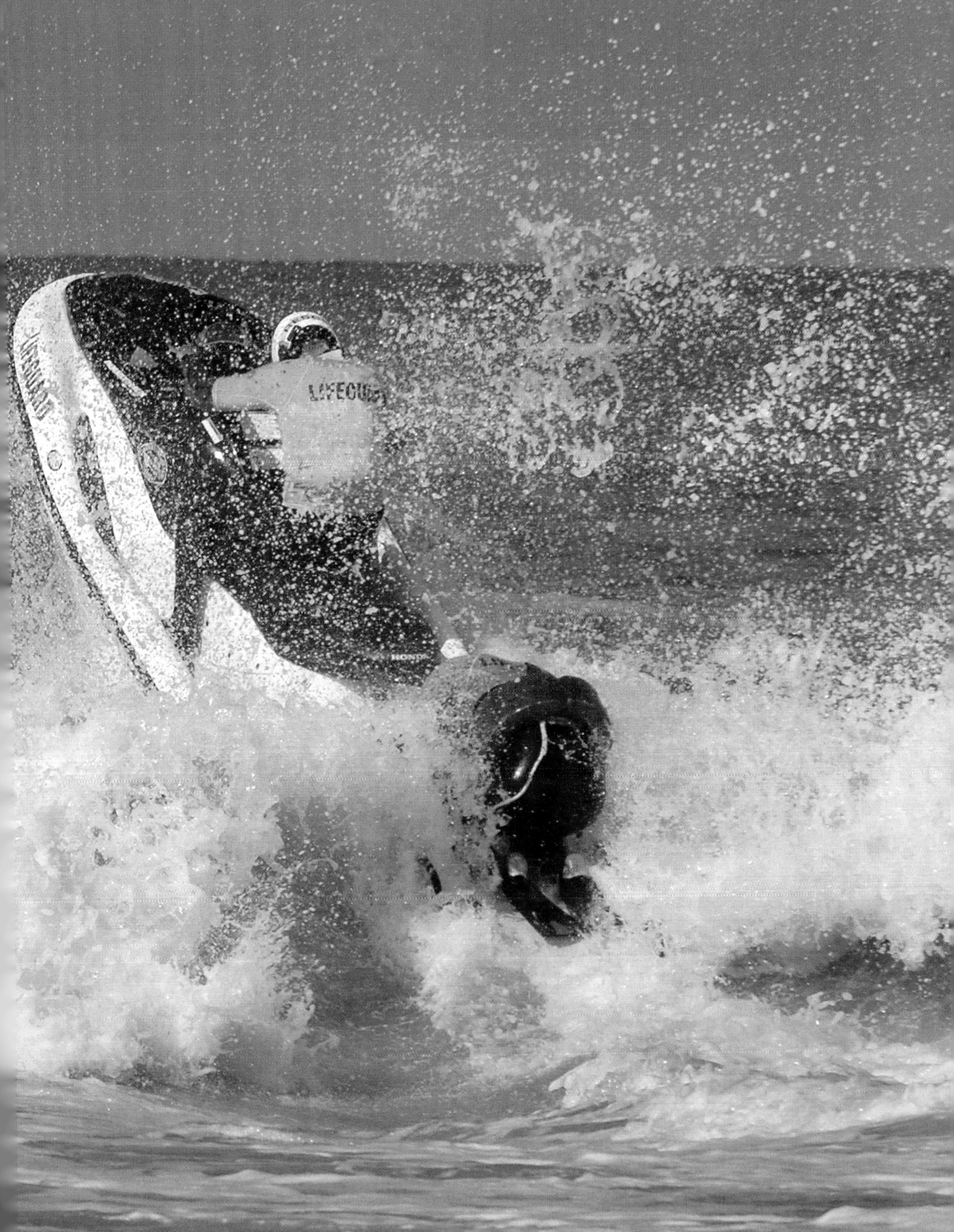

When you see an emergency situation, you must have a determination to act as well as the ability to make decisions and provide first aid until medical personnel arrive on the scene.

LEARNING GOALS

In this chapter you will learn about:

- The chain of survival
- Evaluating situations
- Calling for help
- Providing care
- Primary and secondary surveys

CHAIN OF SURVIVAL

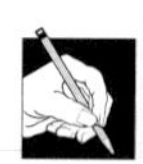

The chain of survival is a necessary sequence of events that must occur when you recognize an emergency situation. The survival and recovery of the victim depends on each step in the sequence taking place in order. You are vital to the chain of survival and responsible for the first three links in the chain. The chain of survival is:

1. Recognize that an emergency exists and evaluate the situation.
2. Call the local emergency number for help.
3. Provide care (CPR, rescue breathing, or first aid) until medical personnel arrive.
4. Emergency medical services (EMS) provide advanced care and transport to a medical facility.
5. The hospital takes over from EMS to provide further treatment.
6. Rehabilitation specialists help the victim return to their previous state of health.

In your aquatic or safety training course (such as scuba diver), you learned that you should stop, think, and then act to resolve any problem or difficulty. With first aid, the first three steps of the chain of survival are very similar. They are:

- Evaluate the situation.
- Call for help.
- Care for the victim.

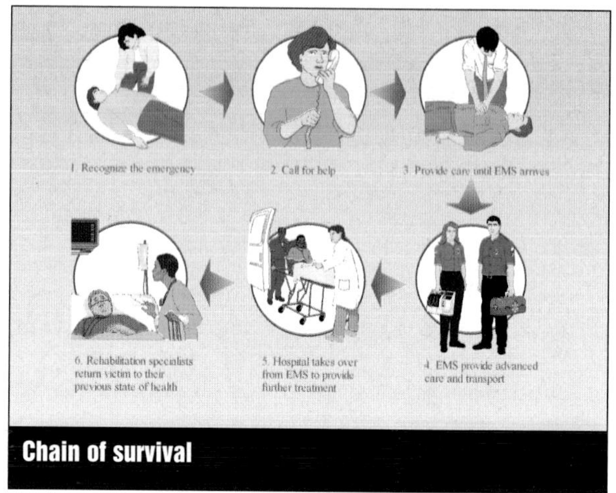

Chain of survival

EVALUATE THE SITUATION

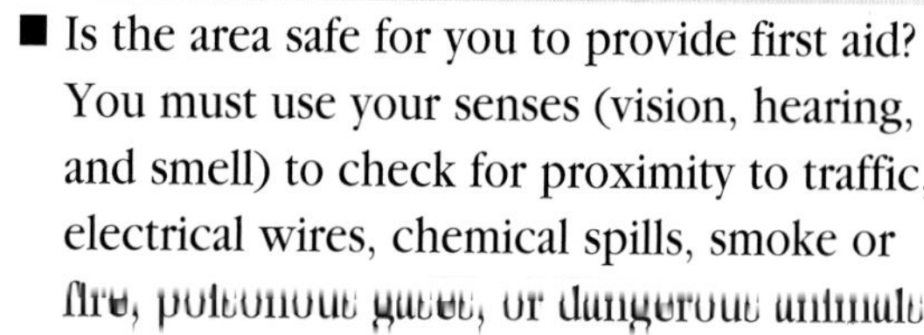

There are a number of questions you must answer in a short time to evaluate the situation.

- Is the area safe for you to provide first aid? You must use your senses (vision, hearing, and smell) to check for proximity to traffic, electrical wires, chemical spills, smoke or fire, poisonous gases, or dangerous animals.
- What appears to have happened? The type of emergency you encounter will determine the treatment you need to give to the victims.
- Are there multiple victims? If you have more than one victim, you must classify them according to injury and rank them by need for care:

- *Critical.* These victims have a life threatening injury or illness that can be corrected or treated successfully.
- *Serious.* These victims do not have life threatening injuries and appear to be stable,

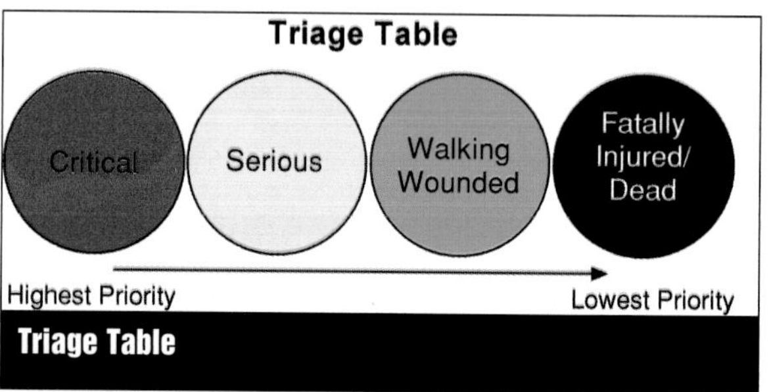

Triage Table

but their condition might worsen if they do not receive care.

- *Walking Wounded.* These victims appear to be stable and can move themselves to a safe location.
- *Fatally Injured or Dead.* These victims have injuries so extreme that it is obvious that they cannot be helped.

Classifying victims in this manner is called triage, and this system enables you to provide care that benefits the greatest number of victims.

■ Is there anyone else close by to help? Even if these people do not know first aid, they can assist you in calling for help or comforting others at the scene. They might also know the cause of the emergency.

CALL FOR HELP

You need to know your local emergency number. It might be 9-1-1, 0 for operator, 1-1-2, or another number. Keep this number posted by your telephone at home and at work.

You must call for emergency help for any of the following situations:

- ■ The victim is unconscious or becomes unconscious.
- ■ The victim has chest pain or pressure.
- ■ The victim is having difficulty breathing.
- ■ The victim is bleeding severely.
- ■ The victim has pain or pressure in their abdomen.
- ■ The victim has slurred speech, a severe headache, or has a seizure.
- ■ The victim has a head, neck, or back injury.
- ■ The victim has broken bones.
- ■ The victim is passing or vomiting blood.
- ■ The victim has been poisoned.
- ■ The victim of drowning or near-downing.

In any other situation, you must use your own best judgment in calling for help. Just remember, when in doubt - call!

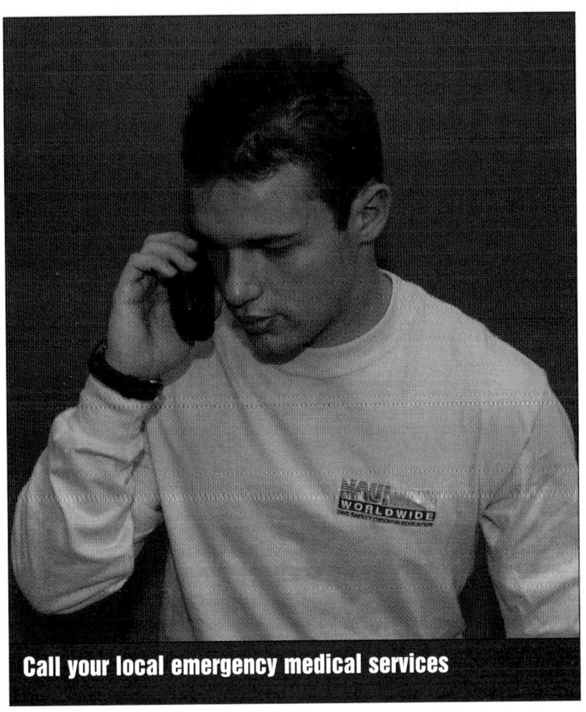

Call your local emergency medical services

CARE FOR THE VICTIM

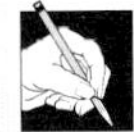

Care or treatment begins with an assessment of the victim. This assessment consists of a primary survey and a secondary survey. Treatment continues until medical personnel arrive to take over the situation.

Primary Survey

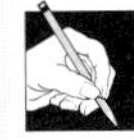

The first step in the primary survey is to determine if the victim is responsive and it is still safe to provide assistance. If the victim does not respond to you, perform the following steps:

1. Check their airway to be sure it is open.
2. Look, listen, and feel for breathing.
3. Check for circulation or any other signs of circulation (coughing or movement).
4. Provide rescue breathing or CPR if necessary.
5. Control any bleeding.
6. Treat for shock.

If the victim responds to you, perform the following steps:

1. Tell them your name.

2. Tell them you know first aid and can help them.
3. Ask them if you can help them. (If a victim refuses assistance you must respect their wishes.)
4. Control any severe bleeding.
5. Determine their level of consciousness, awareness, and orientation. Do they respond to questions? Do they know their name, the date, and where they are?
6. Complete a head-to-toe examination (the secondary survey). If you need to touch the victim, ask their permission.
7. Provide the appropriate first aid.
8. Treat for shock.

Secondary Survey

The secondary survey is also known as the head-to-toe examination. Record your results, including the date, time, victim's name, that permission was given, and anything relevant to the incident. If the victim's condition prevents the performance of one or more of these evaluations, record the omitted item and reason. Provide this written report to EMS or other medical personnel when they arrive on scene. During the secondary survey, you:

1. Ask the victim what happened.
2. Ask the victim how they are feeling.
3. Ask the victim if they feel any pain. If so, where?
4. Ask the victim what led up to the problem (if their problem is medical).
5. Ask the victim if they have a medical condition that might have caused the problem. Ask them if they have taken or skipped their medications.
6. Ask the victim when they last ate.
7. Check the victim's respiration. Count the number of breaths in a minute (or count for 15 seconds and multiply times four) and listen to how they are breathing. Is it rapid, labored, or rasping?

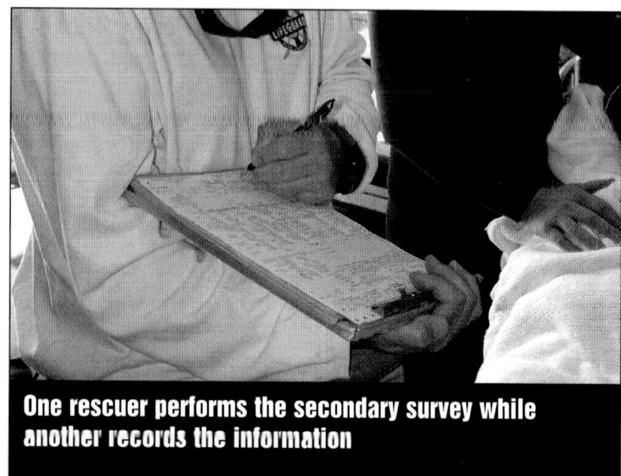

One rescuer performs the secondary survey while another records the information

8. Check the victim's pulse rate. Count the number of beats in a minute (or count for 15 seconds and multiply times four). Is it rapid or slow?
9. Check the victim's skin condition. Is it moist or clammy, hot or cold, flushed or pale?
10. Check the victim's head and neck for signs of injury. Visually check and gently feel for abnormalities, protrusions, or swelling.
11. Check the victim's chest and back for signs of injury. Visually check and gently feel for abnormalities, protrusions, or swelling.
12. Check the victim's abdomen for signs of injury. Visually check and gently feel for abnormalities, protrusions, or swelling. With the victim's permission, you may also gently press with the fingers of one hand on the four quadrants (upper and lower, right and left) of his or her abdomen to check for discomfort or pain.
13. Check the victim's extremities for signs of injury. Visually check and gently feel for abnormalities, protrusions, or swelling.
14. Perform a 5-minute neurological examination if you suspect a scuba diving injury, nervous system (head, neck, spinal cord) injury, or stroke. Use the following steps to perform the examination:

a. **Orientation**. Determine the victim's level of consciousness, awareness, and orientation by how they respond to questions. Ask the victim's name and the current date. Ask the victim if they know where they are. Although the victim might appear to be alert, these questions might reveal confusion.

b. **Eyes**. Have the victim hold their head still. Ask the victim to use their eyes to follow your hand or finger while you move your hand up and down and side to side. Your hand or finger should be about 18 inches (45 cm) from the victim's face. The eyes should track smoothly in all directions and should not jerk from side to side. Check the victim's peripheral vision. Ask the victim to look straight ahead. Move your finger from the side of their head towards the front and have them tell you when it appears in their field of vision. See if the pupils are equal in size and respond to light.

c. **Forehead**. Have the victim close their eyes while you lightly touch their forehead and face. Check that feeling is present and if it is equal on both sides. Have the victim furrow their brow. Note if there is a difference.

d. **Face**. Ask the victim to whistle. Check to see if the victim can pucker their lips. Ask the victim to smile. Note if there is a difference in facial muscles. Ask the victim to clench their teeth. Feel their jaw for equal muscle strength. Check for skin sensation.

e. **Ears**. Ask if their hearing is abnormal. Have the victim close their eyes. Check their hearing by holding your hand about two feet (0.6 meters) away from the victim's ear and rub your thumb and forefinger together. Move your hand closer until they can hear the sound. Repeat for the other ear.

f. **Gag reflex**. Ask the victim to swallow while watching their "Adam's Apple" move up and down.

g. **Tongue**. Ask the victim to stick out their tongue. It should come out straight, in the middle of the mouth.

h. **Shoulders**. Place your hands on the victim's shoulders and ask them to shrug. Note if there is a difference in strength. Check for skin sensation.

i. **Arms**. Have the victim squeeze your fingers. Note if there is a difference in strength. Have the victim grasp their hands together at chest level, with elbows high. Gently push and then pull the elbows while the victim resists the motion. Note if there is a difference in strength. Ask the victim to close their eyes and touch their nose with each forefinger in turn. Check for skin sensation.

j. **Chest**. Have the victim close their eyes. Check for skin sensation.

k. **Lower extremities**. If the victim is ambulatory, have them walk on their heels for a short distance, then turn around and walk back on their toes.

The results of your primary and secondary survey will give you the basic information you need to be able to assist the victim.

REVIEW QUESTIONS

1. The chain of survival is ________________________ that must occur when you recognize an emergency situation.

2. There are a number of questions you must answer in a short time to evaluate the situation. They are: ________________________
____
____
____

3. You must call for emergency help for any of the following situations - list 5 of the 11 examples from the text. ________________________
____
____

4. Care or treatment begins with ________________________.

5. The first step in the primary survey is to determine if the victim is __________ and it is ________________________.

6. The secondary survey is also known as the ________________________.

Notes

CHAPTER 5

Cardiopulmonary Resuscitation (CPR)

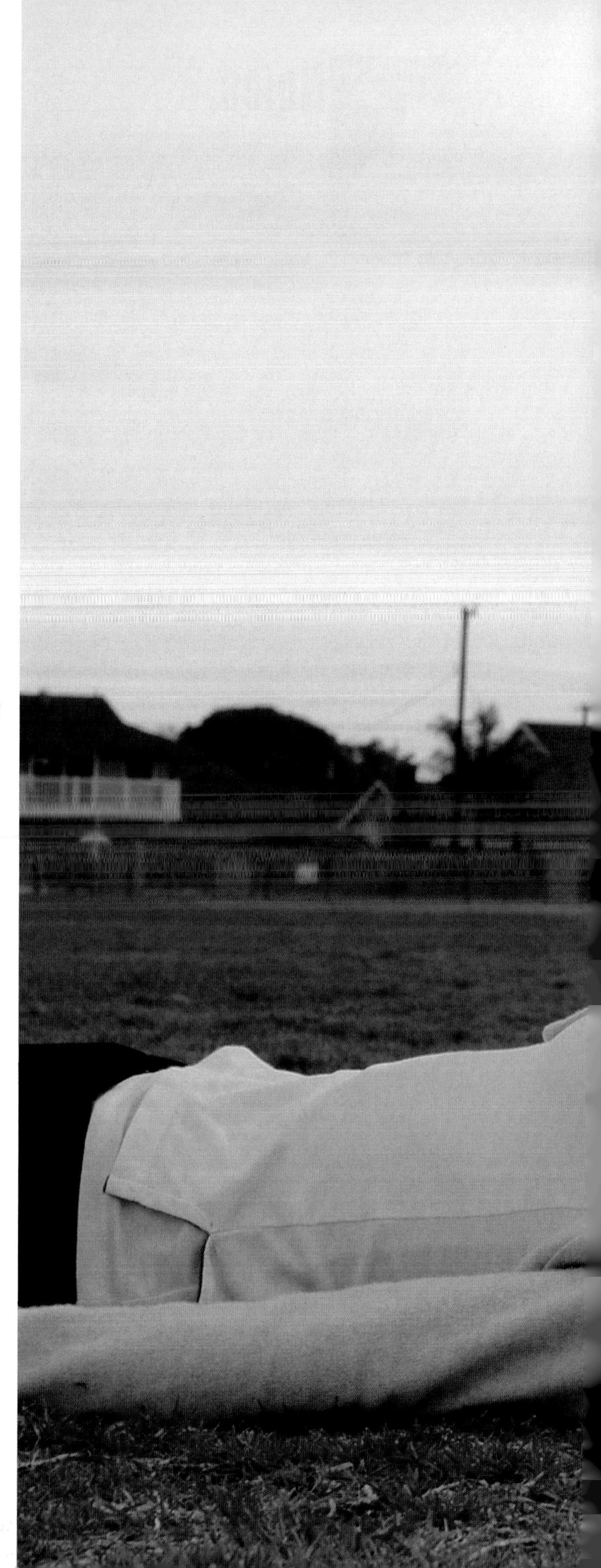

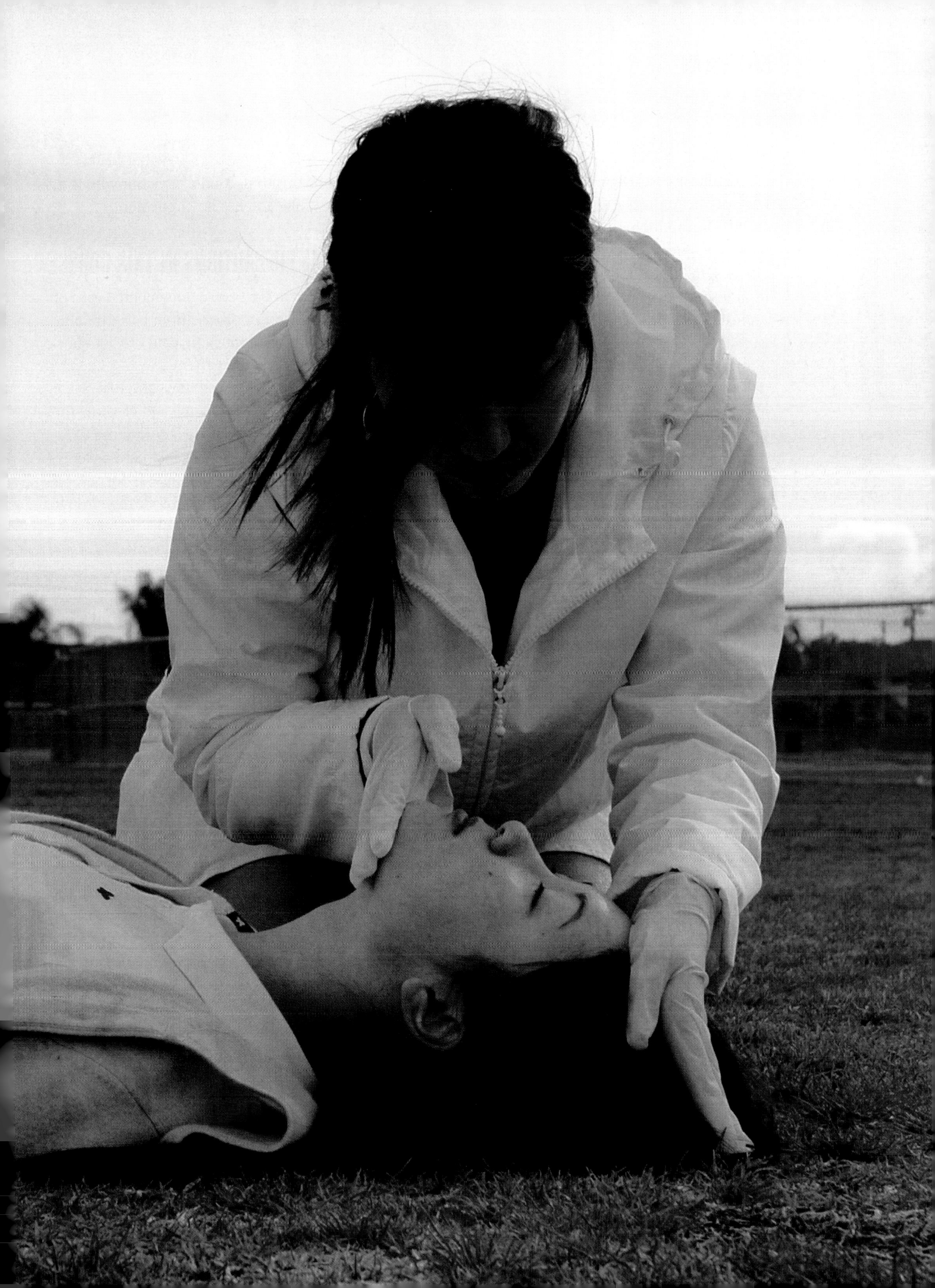

Cardiovascular Disease (CVD) includes both coronary heart disease and strokes. The World Health Organization estimates that each year 16.6 million people worldwide die of cardiovascular diseases. In 2001 there were 7.2 million deaths from heart disease and 5.5 million from stroke. Annual deaths from CVD are projected to surpass 24 million per year by 2030.

Heart disease kills 2 million Europeans every year and is the most common cause of death in the EU. Every year, more than 1 million Americans suffer a heart attack and about 500,000 people die from heart disease. Recent studies indicate that the incidence of heart disease will dramatically increase in the next two decades in the Asia Pacific region to levels that will surpass those in the United States and Europe unless preventive interventions are successfully implemented. The risk factors for heart disease and strokes are similar.

A heart attack, stroke, or drowning, can happen anywhere, at any time, to anyone. Someday you might be called upon to aid a relative, friend, coworker, or even a complete stranger. Knowing CPR and the appropriate actions to take could save that person's life. This chapter will prepare you to know the steps to follow, in an emergency, and to aid the person in distress until they are in the care of medical personnel. For more information on drowning and scuba diving maladies, see "Chapter 18, Water Hazards".

LEARNING GOALS

In this chapter you will learn about:

- Universal precautions as they apply to CPR training and practice
- Risk factors and healthy living
- Heart disease and strokes
- Warning signs of heart attack and stroke
- The steps needed to care for the following people whether they be an adult, child, or infant: a conscious victim of a heart attack or stroke, an unconscious breathing victim, a non-breathing victim, a victim who is not breathing and has no circulation

UNIVERSAL PRECAUTIONS IN THIS COURSE

There has never been a documented case of anyone contracting a disease from using training aids and manikins during a first aid or CPR course. This is according to the CDC.

Your NAUI instructor follows the CDC's Guidelines for decontaminating and cleaning the manikins and training aids used during the CPR course. As long as you follow instructions for decontamination during the course, your risk of contracting any kind of disease is extremely low. Always be sure to wash your hands before and after participating in any class activities. Also, do not eat, drink, or chew gum during class.

You should ask for a separate training manikin if any of the following situations apply to you:

- You have a cold or sore throat.
- You have open sores around your mouth or on your hands
- You have a compromised immune system or condition that makes you unusually prone to getting an infection.
- You know you have a chronic infection such as AIDS, Hepatitis B, or Hepatitis C.
- You have tested positive for HIV antibodies.

You will not be asked to provide an explanation if you ask for a separate training manikin. If you have any medical condition or disability that will prohibit you from participating in any of the physical skill sessions, please let your instructor know. They will make reasonable accommodations to enable you to participate.

RISK FACTORS AND HEALTHY LIVING

Everyone should be concerned with ways to live healthy and prevent heart attacks and strokes. The American Heart Association has identified several risk factors. Some risk factors

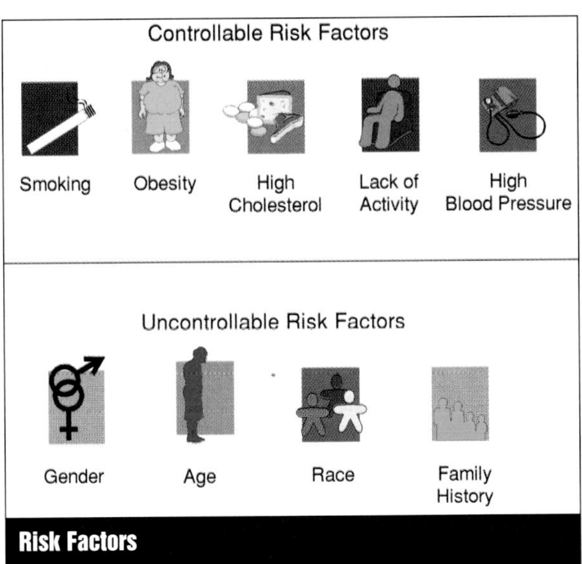

Risk Factors

for heart attacks and strokes are genetic and some are attributed to lifestyle. The more risk factors you have, the greater your chance to develop coronary (heart) disease. The risk factors that are genetic and cannot be changed include:

- Gender. Men have a greater risk of heart attack than women. Men tend to have heart attacks earlier in life. A woman's chance of having a heart attack increases after menopause.
- Age. Eighty-four percent of people who die of coronary heart disease are older than 65. Older women are more likely to die from a heart attack than older men.
- Race. African-Americans have more severe high blood pressure problems than Caucasians and a higher risk of heart disease. Mexican-Americans, Native Americans, Native Hawaiians, and some Asian Americans also have a higher risk of heart disease. This is partly due to higher rates of obesity and diabetes in these groups.
- A family history of heart attack or stroke. Children of parents with heart disease are more likely to develop heart disease. People with a strong family history of heart disease usually have other risk factors.

There are also risk factors that can be controlled or changed. You can help change some of them on your own. Others require the help of your physician to change. The risk factors that can be controlled or changed include:

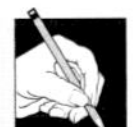

- Smoking. If you don't smoke, don't start. If you do smoke, it's never too late to quit.
- Obesity. The presence of too much body fat helps cause diseases such as heart disease, high blood pressure, diabetes, and gall bladder disease. The best way to lose weight is to limit your calorie intake and increase your output of energy through exercise.
- High cholesterol. Modify your diet to lower your cholesterol level. Eat less saturated fat and substitute low-fat products for high-fat products.
- Lack of physical activity. It's never too late to start some form of physical activity. One suggestion is walking briskly for 20 to 30 minutes, three times a week to exercise your cardiovascular system.
- High blood pressure. Modifying your diet and losing weight are two key ways to help lower your blood pressure. Some people also need to take blood pressure medication prescribed by their physician.

You cannot change your gender, age, race, or family history, but controlling or changing the rest of the risk factors will reduce the chance of developing heart disease. Reducing the risk factors will reduce the chance that you will need to be a recipient of the CPR skills you will learn in the next section. Learning the CPR skills will enable you to help someone else in an emergency. Knowing CPR and the appropriate actions to take could save that person's life.

HEART DISEASE AND STROKES

Cardiac emergencies include angina pectoris (an intense, suffocating pain in the chest) and myocardial infarctions (heart attacks). Angina pectoris is usually caused by atherosclerosis. Atherosclerosis is a condition caused by fatty deposits on the inner lining of the arteries. These deposits restrict the normal blood flow by narrowing the arteries until they are almost or completely blocked. Strokes are the result of an interruption of blood flow to the brain or a hemorrhage from a bleed. Taking a basic first aid course (if you have not already done so) teaches you the procedures to aid those afflicted with these conditions.

Angina Pectoris

People who have atherosclerosis commonly suffer from angina pectoris, which is caused by fatty deposits on the inner lining and a narrowing of the arteries. Angina pectoris is a specific chest discomfort caused by inadequate blood flow through the blood vessels of the heart. It usually occurs when a person overexerts during physical activity and circulation to the heart muscle is compromised by the narrowed arteries. People with advanced disease can have an episode of angina pectoris at rest. People who suffer from angina pectoris usually have nitroglycerine medication to stop the pain associated with angina. The signs and symptoms of angina include:

- Chest pain or a feeling of pressure in the chest that comes and goes
- Nausea and sweating
- Shortness of breath

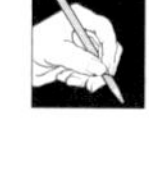

Use the following steps to aid someone suffering from angina:

1. Have the victim stop physical activity.
2. Help the victim rest in a comfortable position.
3. Assist the victim with their medication, if necessary. Do not administer the medication for them.
4. Call for help if their symptoms do not subside or seem to be getting worse.

Myocardial Infarctions (Heart Attack)

Myocardial infarction (MI) occurs when there is death of some of the muscle cells of the heart as a result of a lack of supply of oxygen and other nutrients. This lack of supply is caused by a closure of one of the arteries that supply a particular part of the heart muscle with blood. This occurs most of the time from the process of atherosclerosis in coronary vessels. The signs and symptoms of a heart attack include:

- Pressure or pain in the chest that lasts more than a few minutes
- Pain that spreads to the shoulders, neck, or arms
- Nausea
- Sweating
- Shortness of breath
- Pale or ashen skin
- Lightheadedness

Denial is often associated with the onset of a heart attack. Use the following steps to assist someone having a heart attack:

1. Have the victim stop physical activity.
2. Help the victim rest comfortably, with their upper body slightly elevated.
3. Loosen any tight clothing (with victim's permission, if conscious).
4. Call for help if the symptoms persist for more than a few minutes or worsen.
5. Monitor for breathing and circulation.
6. Be prepared to administer cardiopulmonary resuscitation (CPR).

Stroke

A stroke occurs when there is an interruption of blood flow to the brain , usually from a blood clot in a major artery. Strokes can stem from a thrombus, embolism, or hemorrhage.

A thrombus is a blood clot that forms in a blood vessel. An embolism is a thrombus or other blockage that has moved from the area where it formed to another area of the body. (Arterial gas embolism (AGE) or air embolism is a scuba diving malady in which air has been introduced into the circulatory system by a rupture of lung tissue.) Hemorrhagic strokes occur when a blood vessel bursts within the brain.

Strokes usually occur in older people, but they can occur in people of all ages. People who smoke, have high blood pressure, are obese, have high cholesterol, diabetes, or heart disease are at an increased risk for a stroke. The signs and symptoms of a stroke include:

- A severe headache
- Sudden numbness of the face, an arm, or a leg
- Unexplained dizziness or staggering
- Inability to speak, inability to understand, slurred or incoherent speech or drooping of one side of the face
- Dimness or loss of vision in one eye
- Loss of consciousness

Use the following steps to care for someone you think is having a stroke:

1. Help the victim rest comfortably.
2. Call for help.
3. Comfort the victim. They might not understand what is happening to them.
4. If the victim is unconscious, drooling, or having trouble swallowing, place the victim on their side in the recovery position to help drain fluids from their mouth. See "Recovery Positions" at the end of this chapter.
5. Monitor breathing and circulation.

PERFORMING CPR

In addition to CPR as practiced by healthcare professionals, two levels of CPR skills are recognized: CPR for lay rescuers and CPR for professional rescuers. Because this course may be taught to professional rescuers (such as lifeguards, scuba instructors, divemasters, and public safety officers) as well as to members of the general public, the performance skills for both will be presented.

If you see a person who appears to be unconscious, there are a specific series of steps you must take to start the chain of survival discussed previously. Here you will learn the steps for providing CPR for adults, children, and infants (newborn to 1 year old).

RESPONSE SEQUENCE

When you see a person who appears to be unconscious or witness a victim of sudden collapse, you must respond quickly and appropriately. First, survey the scene for safety. Your next action is to determine if the person is unconscious by gently shaking them and asking if they are okay. If the victim is unresponsive, shout for help if none is present.

For an unresponsive adult, the lay rescuer should immediately send someone to activate the emergency response system and retrieve an AED (automated external defibrillator) if one is available and the rescuer is trained in its use. If the rescuer is all alone, they should call the emergency response system, retrieve the AED, and then return to the victim to open the airway, check for breathing, and provide appropriate care.

For an unresponsive child or infant, the lone lay rescuer should open the airway and check for breathing. If none is present, the rescuer should provide 5 cycles of CPR (about 2 minutes-see "Child Life Support", below) before leaving the victim to activate the emergency response system and retrieve the AED.

For the professional rescuer or healthcare provider, the response sequence is similar, with a few differences.

If the lone professional rescuer witnesses the sudden collapse of a victim of any age, they should verify non-responsiveness of the victim, then immediately activate the emergency response system, retrieve an AED if available, then begin CPR and use of the AED.

If the professional rescuer is rescuing an unresponsive infant or child or a victim of drowning or other asphyxial cause of arrest, the rescuer should provide 5 cycles of CPR (about 2 minutes) before leaving the victim to activate the emergency response system and retrieve the AED.

ADULT BASIC LIFE SUPPORT

Adult basic life support begins with the following actions:

- Positioning the victim
- Opening the airway
- Checking for breathing

Then, based on your findings at each step, you provide the proper care. You do not provide rescue breathing if the victim begins to breathe spontaneously when you open their airway. You do not start CPR if the victim is breathing. You only start CPR if the victim is not breathing (ignoring occasional, noisy gasps).

Positioning

Before you can start checking for airway and breathing, you must position the victim correctly. They might be lying face down or slumped in a sitting position. Whenever you position a victim, always be aware of the possibility of a neck or head injury. When positioning a victim, be sure to support their head and neck and keep it in a straight line with their back. You must position the victim to be lying on a flat, hard surface and on their back.

Open the Airway

Before you can assess whether a victim is breathing, you must open their airway using the head-tilt, chin-lift method. Use the following steps to open an adult's airway:

1. Place one hand on the victim's forehead.
2. Place the forefinger and middle finger of

The following is a summary of the evidence-based recommendations for the performance of basic life support from the 2005 Consensus Conference:

Rescuers begin CPR if the victim is unconscious, not moving, and not breathing (ignoring occasional gasps).

For mouth-to-mouth ventilation or for bag-valve-mask ventilation with room air or oxygen, the rescuer should deliver each breath in 1 second and should see visible chest rise.

Increased emphasis on the process of CPR: push hard at a rate of 100 compressions per minute, allow full chest recoil, and minimize interruptions in chest compressions.

For the single rescuer of an infant (except newborns), child, or adult victim, use a single compression-ventilation ratio of 30:2 to simplify teaching, promote skills retention, increase the number of compressions given, and decrease interruptions in compressions. During 2-rescuer CPR of the infant or child, healthcare providers should use a 15:2 compression-ventilation ratio.

During CPR for a patient with an advanced airway (ie, tracheal tube, esophageal-tracheal combitube [Combitube], laryngeal mask airway [LMA]) in place, deliver ventilations at a rate of 8 to 10 per minute for infants (excepting neonates), children and adults, without pausing during chest compressions to deliver the ventilations.

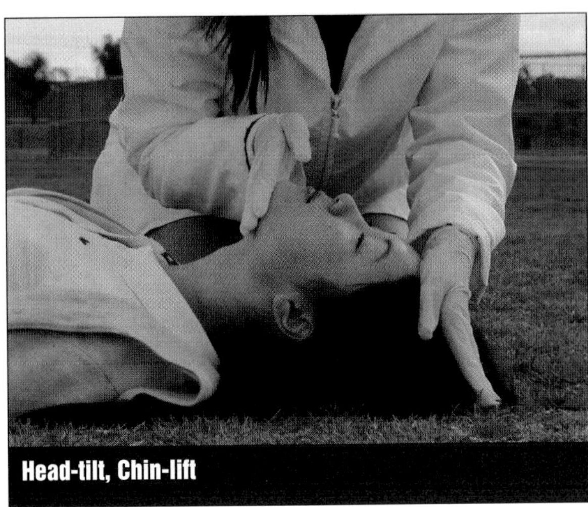
Head-tilt, Chin-lift

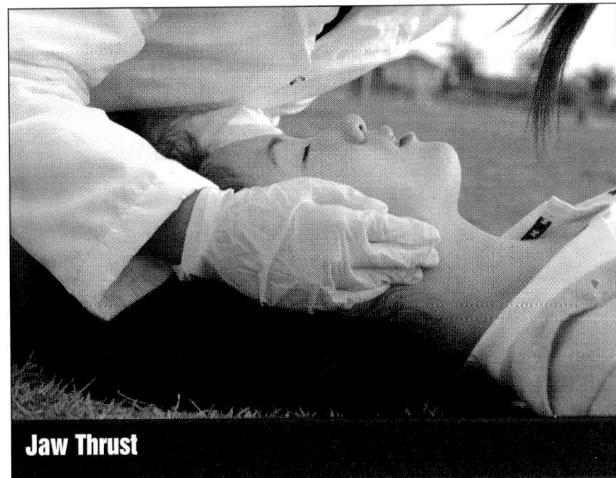
Jaw Thrust

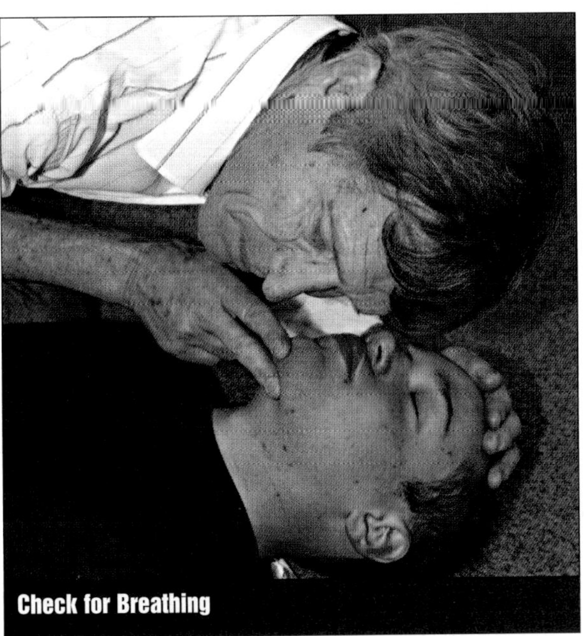
Check for Breathing

your other hand on the bony part of the victim's chin. Avoid the soft area under the jaw.

3. Use both hands to gently tilt the head backward. Do not close the victim's mouth.

If you have reason to suspect a cervical spine injury, use the following steps for a modified jaw thrust without a head-tilt:

1. Position yourself behind or at the side of the victim's head.
2. Place your hands on both sides of the victim's head and place your fingers gently along the back edge of the bone on both sides of the jaw.
3. Place your thumbs on the front of the upper jaw bone near the cheeks.
4. Pull up with your fingers to gently move the victim's lower jaw away from the upper jaw to open the mouth and airway.
5. If life-threatening airway obstruction persists, gently tilt the head backward until the airway is open.

The victim might not be breathing because the relaxed tongue has fallen back and blocked the airway. The head tilt, chin lift or the modified jaw thrust raises the tongue, and the victim might begin breathing spontaneously.

Check for Breathing

Once you have the airway open, you must check for breathing. Use the following steps to check for breathing. With your cheek close to the victim's face:

1. Look at the person's chest to see if it is rising and falling.
2. Listen at the victim's nose and mouth to hear air going into and coming out of their airway.
3. Feel for air on your cheek as you are listening.
4. Check for breathing for five seconds. If the victim is breathing, place them in the recovery position and monitor the victim until help arrives.

If you do not see, hear, or feel any evidence of breathing, you must start CPR.

Beginning CPR: Rescue Breaths

Provide two rescue breaths. Use a face shield or barrier mask if possible. Use the following steps to perform rescue breathing:

1. Open the airway using the previously described steps.
2. Pinch the victim's nose at the fleshy part of the nose to close it.
3. Inhale deeply.
4. Seal your lips around the victim's mouth. If available, you should always use a barrier shield or pocket mask between you and the victim.
5. Exhale into the victim's mouth for one second.
6. Watch for the victim's chest to rise as you exhale into their mouth.
7. Move your mouth away from the victim's mouth
8. Inhale deeply.
9. Watch for the victim's chest to fall
10. Give a second breath. Exhale into the victim's mouth for one second. (For children, infants, and known drowning victims give an additional three initial breaths-for a total of five breaths.)

If you are not able to deliver breaths to the victim, you may not have opened the airway properly. Reposition the head to reopen the airway as described above and try again.

After the initial rescue breaths, look for normal breathing or movement by the victim in response to the breaths. If normal breathing returns, place the victim in the recovery position and monitor them until help arrives.

If breathing does not return when you open the airway, the lay rescuer should move directly to cardiopulmonary resuscitation (CPR) and begin cycles of chest compressions and ventilations as explained in the following pages.

The professional rescuer should attempt to feel a pulse (see "Checking for a Pulse"). If a pulse is felt, the professional rescuer should provide rescue breathing. If no pulse is felt, the rescuer should proceed to CPR cycles of chest compressions and ventilations.

FOR PROFESSIONAL RESCUERS AND NAUI DIVERS RESPONDING TO DROWNING VICTIMS

Checking for a Pulse

After giving initial rescue breaths, the professional rescuer or healthcare provider must check the victim for circulation. Check for a pulse for no more than 10 seconds. Use the following steps to check for a pulse:

1. Place your index finger and middle finger on the victim's Adam's apple.
2. Slide your fingers towards you and down into the groove on the victim's neck.
3. Feel for a pulse in the carotid artery for no more than 10 seconds.

If you do not feel a pulse, you will need to perform cardiopulmonary resuscitation (CPR) as explained below. If you do feel a pulse, continue to provide rescue breathing without chest compressions.

Rescue Breathing

1. If the victim has a pulse, continue with rescue breathing. Open the airway and close the victim's nose using the steps described above.
2. Administer one breath every 5 seconds.
3. After about 1 minute (12 breath cycles), check for a pulse again, as explained above in Checking for a Pulse.
4. Continue rescue breathing until help arrives or until the victim begins to breathe on their own. Continue to check for a

pulse every so often. If a pulse is no longer detected, begin chest compressions.

If the victim vomits, roll them onto their side and clear the mouth and throat of vomit before continuing.

If the victim has an injury to their mouth and you cannot breathe through their mouth, you can seal their lips and breathe through their nose instead. Be sure to seal your lips completely around their nose.

If the victim has had a tracheotomy and has a stoma (a permanent opening) in their neck, you can close their mouth and nose and breathe through the stoma. Be sure to seal your lips completely around the stoma.

One-Person CPR

If a person is not breathing (ignoring occasional gasps), you must perform CPR. Use the following steps to perform CPR on an adult:

1. Envision an imaginary line between the nipples and then place the heel of your dominant hand on the sternum (breastbone) just below the line, or more simply, in the center of the chest.
2. Place the other hand on top of the hand on the sternum.
3. Interlock or lift your fingers so no fingers are directly touching the chest.
4. Have your shoulders directly over your hands on the victim's chest and lock your elbows.
5. Perform 30 chest compressions at a rate of 100 compressions per minute. Push straight down on the breastbone for 1.5 to 2 inches (4 to 5 centimeters) with each compression. Count as you compress - 1 and 2 and 3 and 4 and 5 and…and 30.
6. Stop compressions and administer 2 rescue breaths.
7. Return your hands to the correct position on the victim's chest and give another 30 compressions.
8. Continue the cycle of 30 compressions and 2 breaths until the victim revives, help arrives to take over, you are too exhausted to continue, or a physician tells you to stop. Stop to recheck the victim only if they start breathing on their own.

If the victim vomits, roll them onto their side and clear the mouth and throat of vomit before continuing.

If signs of recovery are present after any cycle, position the victim on their side in the recovery position and monitor for breathing and circulation. See "Recovery Position" at the end of this chapter. If trained to do so, adminster supplemental oxygen, if available.

FOR PROFESSIONAL RESCUERS AND HEALTHCARE PROFESSIONALS

Two-Person CPR

All professional rescuers (healthcare professionals, EMS personnel, and laypersons who have a duty to respond in an emergency) should know two-person CPR. In two-person CPR, the rescuers position themselves as follows:

- Rescuer one is positioned at the victim's head to keep the airway open, provide rescue breathing, and monitor for signs of breathing and circulation.
- Rescuer two is positioned at the victim's side to perform chest compressions.

Use the following steps to perform two-person CPR:

1. Rescuer one opens the airway and checks for breathing.
2. Rescuer one administers two rescue breaths. If a mask with attached breathing bag is available, use it to administer the rescue breaths. Be sure to hold the mask firmly against the victim's face to form a seal.

3. Rescuer one checks for signs of circulation for no more than 10 seconds as described previously in "Checking a Pulse".
4. Rescuer two starts chest compressions if no signs of circulation can be determined. Thirty compressions are delivered at a rate of 100 compressions per minute. Push straight down on the breastbone for 1.5 to 2 inches (4 to 5 centimeters) with each compression. Count as you compress - 1 and 2 and 3 and 4 and 5… and 30.
5. Rescuer one administers two rescue breaths at the end of the 30 compressions.
6. Continue the cycle until the victim revives or help arrives to take over.

Before rescuer two becomes fatigued, the two rescuers should switch positions. Switch positions about every two minutes. The switch takes place between sets of compressions, immediately after rescue breaths are given. The switch should be made as quickly as possible with minimal interruption of chest compressions.

NOTE: In two person CPR for children and infants, the compression to ventilation ratio should be changed to 15 compressions to 2 breaths.

CHILD LIFE SUPPORT

For purposes of child life support, anyone between one and eight years old is considered a child. Children usually weigh between 10 kilograms (22 pounds) and 25 kilograms (55 pounds).

Children between the age of one and eight years old generally do not suffer from cardiac disease. Cardiac arrest in a child is usually the result of progressive shock or respiratory failure. CPR for children might be required when there is an injury, an airway obstruction by a foreign object, a drowning, smoke inhalation, or infection. Child life support consists of the following actions:

- Positioning the victim
- Opening the airway
- Checking for breathing

Then, based on your findings at each step, you provide the proper treatment. When treating a child, provide care for one minute before calling for help. Then continue care until help arrives.

Positioning

Before you can start checking for airway, breathing, and circulation, you must position the victim correctly. They might be lying face down or slumped in a sitting position. Whenever you position a victim, always be aware of the possibility of a neck or head injury. When positioning a victim, be sure to support their head and neck and keep it in a straight line with their back. You must position the victim to be lying on a flat, hard surface and on their back.

Open the Airway

Before you can assess whether a victim is breathing, you must open their airway using the head tilt, chin lift method. Use the following steps to open a child's airway:

1. Place one hand on the victim's forehead.
2. Place the forefinger and middle finger of your other hand on the bony part of the victim's chin. Avoid the soft spot under the jaw.
3. Use both hands to gently tilt the head backward. Do not close the victim's mouth.

If you have reason to suspect a cervical spine injury, use the following steps for a modified jaw thrust without head tilt:

1. Position yourself behind the victim's head.
2. Place your hands on both sides of the victim's head and place your fingers gently along the back edge of the bone on both sides of the jaw.
3. Place your thumbs on the front of the upper jaw bone near the cheeks.
4. Pull up with your fingers to gently move the victim's lower jaw away from the

upper jaw to open the mouth and airway.

5. If life-threatening airway obstruction persists, gently tilt the head backward until the airway is open.

Check for Breathing

Once you have the airway open, you must check for breathing. Use the following steps to check for breathing. With your cheek close to the victim's face:

1. Look at the child's chest to see if it is rising and falling.
2. Listen at the victim's nose and mouth to hear air going into and coming out of their airway.
3. Feel for air on your cheek as you are listening.

Check for breathing for five seconds. If the child is breathing, place them on their side in the recovery position and monitor them for continued breathing. See "Recovery Position" at the end of this chapter.

If breathing does not return when you open the airway, or if the child is making irregular gasps, check in the mouth for a foreign object that might be blocking the airway. If you see an object, insert your little finger in the victim's mouth and carefully sweep your finger from one side of the mouth to the other to remove the object. Then recheck for breathing before continuing.

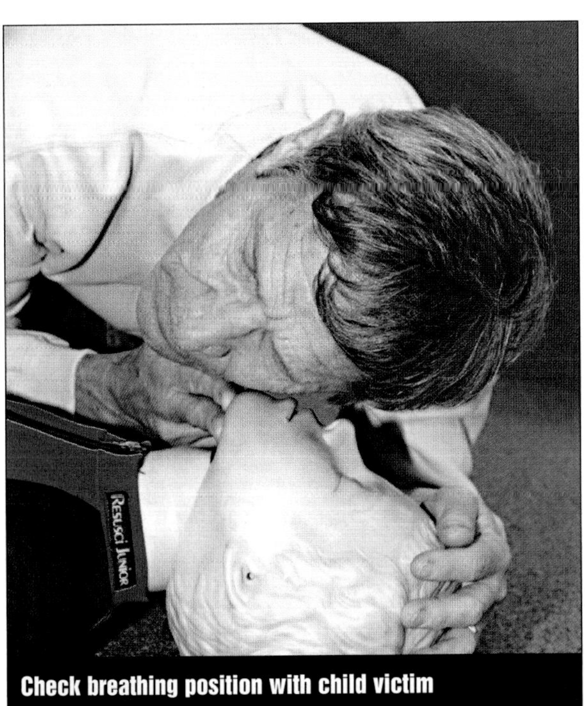
Check breathing position with child victim

If breathing still does not return, you must start CPR.

Beginning CPR: Rescue Breaths

If you do not see, hear, or feel any evidence of breathing, provide two rescue breaths. Use a face shield or barrier mask if possible.

Use the following steps to perform rescue breaths on a child:

1. Open the airway using the previously described steps.
2. Pinch the victim's nose at the fleshy part of the nose to close it.
3. Inhale deeply.
4. Seal your lips around the victim's mouth. If available, you should always use a barrier shield or pocket mask between you and the victim.
5. Exhale into the victim's mouth for one second.
6. Watch for the victim's chest to rise as you exhale into their mouth.
7. Move your mouth away from the victim's mouth.
8. Inhale deeply.
9. Watch for the victim's chest to fall.
10. Give a second breath as described above.

If you are not able to deliver breaths to the victim, you may not have opened the airway properly. Reposition the head to reopen the airway as described above and try again. With children, it may be necessary to reopen the airway several times and move the head through a range of positions to obtain an open airway.

After the initial rescue breaths, check for return of normal breathing or other signs of circulation, such as coughing or movement by the victim. If breathing does not return, but you are certain that there are other signs of circulation, continue with rescue breathing. If there are no signs of circulation or if you are unsure, the lay rescuer should move directly to cardiopulmonary resuscitation (CPR) and begin cycles of chest compressions and ventilations as explained below.

The professional rescuer should attempt to feel a pulse (see "Checking for a Pulse"). If a pulse is felt, the professional rescuer should provide rescue breathing. If no pulse is felt, the rescuer should proceed to CPR cycles of chest compressions and ventilations.

FOR PROFESSIONAL RESCUERS AND HEALTHCARE PROVIDERS

Checking for a Pulse

After giving two initial rescue breaths, the professional rescuer or healthcare provider must check the victim for circulation. Check for a pulse for no more than 10 seconds. Use the following steps to check for a pulse:

1. Place your index finger and middle finger on the victim's Adam's apple.
2. Slide your fingers towards you and down into the groove on the victim's neck.
3. Feel for a pulse in the carotid artery for no more than 10 seconds.

If you do not feel a pulse, you will need to perform cardiopulmonary resuscitation (CPR) as explained below. If you do feel a pulse, continue to provide rescue breathing without chest compressions.

Rescue Breathing for a Child

1. If the victim has signs of circulation, continue with rescue breathing. Open the airway, close the victim's nose, and administer rescue breaths using the steps described above.
2. Administer one breath every 3 seconds.
3. After about 1 minute (20 breath cycles), reassess the victim. Check for signs of circulation as explained above.
4. Continue rescue breathing until help arrives or until the victim begins to breathe on their own.

Child CPR

If a child is not breathing and has no signs of circulation, you must perform CPR. Use the following steps:

1. Envision an imaginary line between the nipples and then place the heel of either hand on the sternum (breastbone) just below the line or more simply in the center of the chest. Do not let your fingers touch the chest.
2. Have your shoulder directly over your hand on the victim's chest and lock your elbow.
3. Perform 30 compressions at a rate of 100 compressions per minute. Push straight down on the breastbone approximately 1/3 to 1/2 the depth of the chest with each compression. Count as you compress - 1 and 2 and 3 and 4 and 5... and 30.
4. Stop compressions and administer 2 rescue breaths.
5. Complete 5 cycles of compressions and rescue breaths (about 2 minutes) before ceasing compressions to activate the emergency response system and/or retrieve an AED.
6. Use the AED or continue CPR at a ratio of 30 compressions to 2 breaths until the victim revives or help arrives to take over.

If signs of recovery are present after any cycle, take the following action:

- Roll the victim onto their left side into the recovery position and monitor for breathing and circulation. If trained to do so, adminster supplemental oxygen, if available.

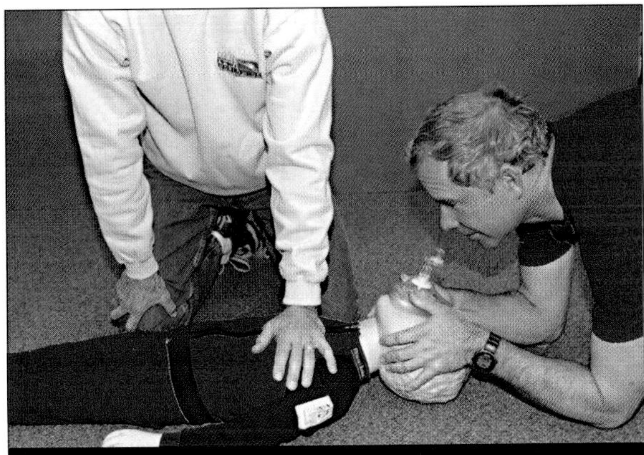

Place heel of hand on the sternum and perform 30 compressions.

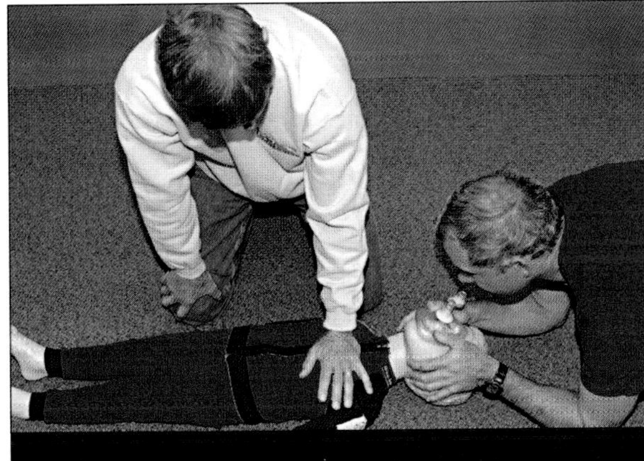

Stop compressions and administer 2 rescue breaths.

INFANT LIFE SUPPORT

For purposes of infant life support, anyone between a newborn and one year old is considered an infant. They usually weigh between 3.5 kilograms (7.7 pounds) and 7 kilograms (15.4 pounds).

Infants generally do not suffer from cardiac disease. Cardiac arrest in an infant is usually the result of progressive shock or respiratory failure. CPR for infants might be required in the case of sudden infant death syndrome, an injury, an airway obstruction by a foreign object, a near drowning, smoke inhalation, or infection. Infant life support consists of the following actions:

- Positioning the victim
- Opening the airway
- Checking for breathing
- Checking for circulation

Then, based on your findings at each step, you provide the proper care. When treating an infant, provide care for one minute before calling for help. Then continue care until help arrives.

Positioning

Before you can start checking for airway, breathing, and circulation, you must position the victim correctly. Whenever you position a victim, always be aware of the possibility of a neck or head injury. When positioning a victim, be sure to support their head and neck and keep it in a straight line with their back. You must position the victim to be lying on a flat, hard surface and on their back.

Open the Airway

Before you can assess whether a victim is breathing, you must open their airway using the head-tilt, chin-lift method. Use the following steps to open an infant's airway:

1. Place one hand on the victim's forehead.
2. Place your forefinger and middle finger of your other hand on the bony part of the victim's chin. Avoid the soft spot under the jaw.
3. Use both hands to gently tilt the head backward. Do not overextend the infant's neck, as the airway is small and flexible and can be collapsed by overextending the neck.

Check for Breathing

Once you have the airway open, you must check for breathing. Use the following steps to check for breathing. With your cheek close to the victim's face:

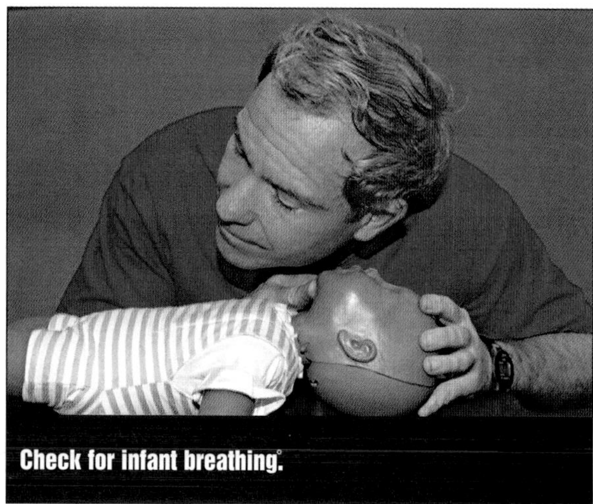
Check for infant breathing.

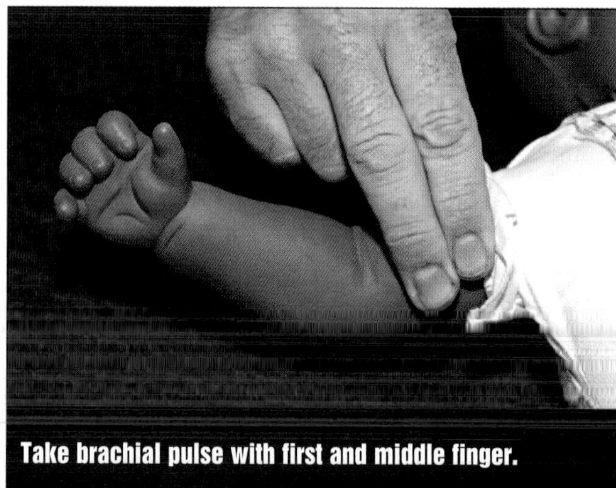
Take brachial pulse with first and middle finger.

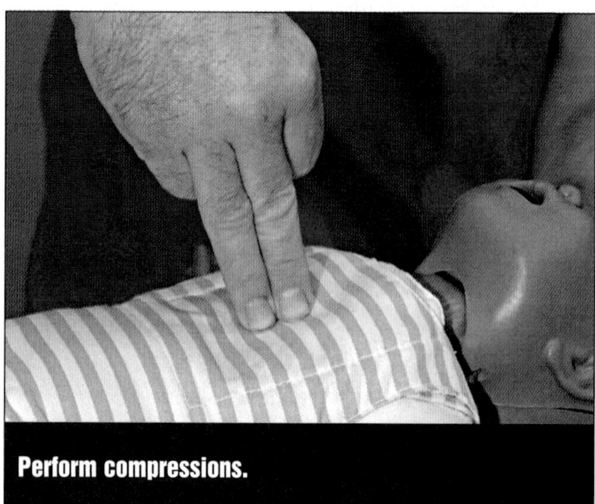
Perform compressions.

1. Look at the infant's chest to see if it is rising and falling.
2. Listen at the victim's nose and mouth to hear air going into and coming out of their airway.
3. Feel for air on your cheek as you are listening.

If breathing does not return when you open the airway, or if the infant is making irregular gasps, check in the mouth for a foreign object that might be blocking the airway. If you see an object, insert your little finger in the victim's mouth and carefully sweep your finger from one side of the mouth to the other to remove the object. Then recheck for breathing before continuing.

Beginning CPR: Rescue Breaths

If you do not see, hear, or feel any evidence of breathing, provide two rescue breaths. Use a face shield or barrier mask if possible. Use the following steps to perform rescue breaths on an infant:

1. Open the airway again using the steps in previously described in "Open the Airway."
2. Inhale.
3. Seal your lips around the victim's mouth and nose. If available, use a barrier shield or pocket mask between you and the victim.
4. Gently exhale into the victim's mouth and nose. With an infant, this should be only a small puff of air, about as much as is in your puffed-up cheeks.
5. Watch for the victim's chest to rise as you exhale into their mouth and nose.
6. Move your mouth away from the victim's face.
7. Inhale.
8. Watch for the victim's chest to fall.
9. Give a second breath. Gently exhale into the victim's mouth and nose.

If you are not able to deliver breaths to the victim, you may not have opened the airway properly. Reposition the head to reopen the airway as described above and try again. With infants, it may be necessary to reopen the airway several times and move the head through a range of positions to obtain an open airway. Avoid tipping the head too far as this may close off the airway.

Check for Circulation

After giving two initial rescue breaths, you must check the victim for circulation. After the initial rescue breaths, look for normal breathing, coughing, or movement by the victim in response to the breaths. If you do not see signs of circulation, you will need to perform cardiopulmonary resuscitation (CPR) as explained in the following steps.

FOR PROFESSIONAL RESCUERS AND HEALTHCARE PROVIDERS

Checking for a Pulse

Healthcare providers must also check for a pulse. Check for a pulse for 5 to 10 seconds. Use the following steps to check for a pulse:

1. Place your index finger and middle finger inside the arm midway between the armpit and the elbow and press the brachial artery against the bone.
2. Feel for a pulse in the brachial artery for 5 to 10 seconds.

If you do not feel a pulse, you will need to perform cardiopulmonary resuscitation (CPR) as explained in the following steps. If you do feel a pulse, continue with rescue breathing and check periodically to see if the victim still has a pulse.

Rescue Breathing for an Infant

1. If the victim has signs of circulation, continue with rescue breathing. Open the airway, and administer rescue breaths using the steps described above.
2. Administer one breath every 3 seconds.
3. After about 1 minute (20 breath cycles), reassess the victim. Check for signs of circulation as explained above.
4. Continue rescue breathing until help arrives or until the victim begins to breathe on their own.

Infant CPR

If an infant is not breathing and has no signs of circulation, you must perform CPR. Use the following steps:

1. Draw an imaginary line connecting the infant's nipples. Place your index finger, middle finger, and ring finger just below the line.
2. Raise your index finger, leaving the other two fingers on the chest. (For two rescuers see the alternative compression method inset.)
3. Perform 30 compressions at a rate of at least 100 compressions per minute. Push straight down on the breastbone approximately 1/3 to 1/2 the depth of the chest with each compression. Count as you compress - 1 and 2 and 3 and 4 and 5… 30.
4. Stop compressions and administer two rescue breaths as previously described.
5. Complete 5 cycles of compressions and rescue breaths (about two 2 minutes) before ceasing compressions to call for help.
6. Continue the cycle until the victim revives or help arrives to take over.

If signs of circulation are present after any cycle, take one of the following actions:

- If the victim is breathing on their own, place them in the recovery position for infants and monitor for breathing and circulation. See "Recovery Position" at the end of this chapter. If trained to do so, administer supplemental oxygen, if available.
- If the victim is not breathing on their own, continue rescue breathing at a rate of 20 breaths per minute. Monitor for signs of breathing every few minutes.

RECOVERY POSITION

A person who is breathing but is unconscious or semiconscious should be placed on their side in the recovery position. The recovery position helps keep the airway open and allows fluids, such as vomit, to drain from the mouth so that they will not be inhaled.

There are several slight variations of the recovery position and several techniques have been suggested to move the victim into it. To place a person in the recovery position, do the following:

- Kneel beside the victim.
- Place the arm nearest you straight out from the body with the elbow bent up as though they were signaling traffic to stop.
- Bring the far arm over and position the back of the hand against the victim's cheek.
- With the other hand, grab the victim's far leg at the knee and bend it up.
- Protecting the victim's head by keeping their hand pressed against the cheek, pull the far knee over towards you to roll the victim onto their side.
- Rest the victim's knee on the ground and adjust their leg so that it stabilizes them on their side. Tilt their head back slightly to make sure that the airway is open. Adjust the hand under their cheek if necessary.
- Monitor the victim.

For an infant, use a modified position to promote an open airway. Drape the infant face down over your forearm with the head slightly lower than the body. Support the infant's head and neck with your hand, being careful not to obstruct the mouth or nose. Alternatively, lay the baby on its side with the head tilted down slightly, and use a pillow or rolled blanket positioned behind the back to maintain the position.

Precautions:

- Do not use the recovery position if you suspect any spinal injury. Use the jaw thrust technique to maintain an open airway.
- A person with a chest injury, such as a pneumothorax or collapsed lung, should be placed with the injured side down so that the good lung is not compressed against the ground.
- A pregnant woman should always be placed on her left side to prevent compression by the fetus and uterus of her inferior vena cava (the major vein that returns blood from the lower body to the heart).

QUICK REFERENCE FOR LIFE SUPPORT

Here is a review of the basic steps of life support:

1. Determine responsiveness by asking the victim if they are okay or tapping them.
2. Call for help if there is no response for an adult. For an infant or child, provide care for two minutes and then call for help.
3. Open the airway.
4. Check for breathing and perform rescue breaths if necessary.
5. Check for signs of circulation (depending on level of training) and perform CPR if necessary.

The following table summarizes the different techniques and rates for respirations and compressions for adults, children, and infants.

Maneuver	Adult	Child	Infant
Airway	Head tilt-chin lift (HCP: suspected trauma, use jaw thrust)		
Breathing Initial	2 breaths at 1 second/breath	2 effective breaths at 1 second/breath	
HCP: Rescue breathing without chest compressions	10 to 12 breaths/min (approximate)	12 to 20 breaths/min (approximate)	
HCP: Rescue breaths for CPR with advanced airway	8 to 10 breaths/min (approximate)		
Foreign-body airway obstruction	Abdominal thrusts		Backslaps and chest thrusts
Circulation HCP: Pulse check (< 10 sec)	Carotid		Brachial or femoral
Compression landmarks	Lower half of sternum, between nipples		Just below nipple line (lower half of sternum)
Compression method Push hard and fast Allow complete recoil	Heel of one hand, other hand on top	Heel of one hand or as for adults	2 or 3 fingers HCP (2 rescuers): 2 thumb-encircling hands
Compression depth	1 1/2 to 2 inches (3.8 to 2 cm)	Approximately one third to one half the depth of the chest	
Compression rate	Approximately 100/min		
Compression-ventilation ratio	30:2 (one or two rescuers)	30:2 (single rescuer) HCP: 15:2 (2 rescuers)	
Defibrillation AED	Use adult pads	Use AED after 5 cycles of CPR (out of hospital). Use pediatric system for child 1 to 8 years if available. HCP: For sudden collapse (oput of hospital) or in hospital arrest use AED as soon as available.	No recommendation for infants <1 year of age.

Note: Maneuvers used by only Healthcare Providers are indicated by "HCP."

REVIEW QUESTIONS

1. The risk factors that can be controlled or changed include: - list 4 of 5 risk factors from the text.

2. Use the following steps to aid someone suffering from angina:

3. Myocardial infarction (MI) occurs when

4. Use the following steps to assist someone having a heart attack:

5. A stroke occurs when

6. The signs and symptoms of a stroke include:

7. Use the following steps to perform CPR on an adult:

8. Use the following steps to perform two-person CPR:

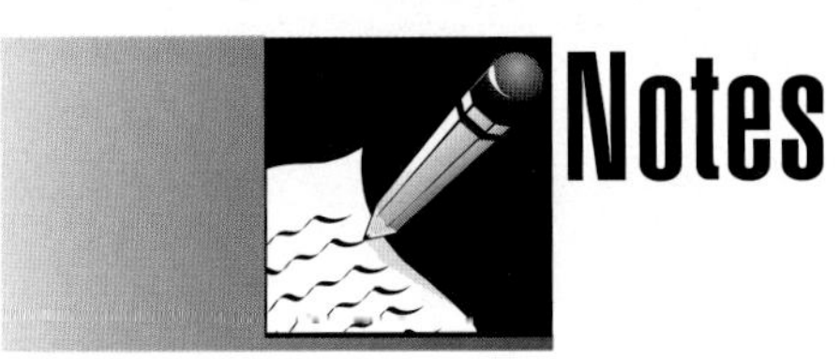

Notes

CHAPTER 6

Foreign Body Airway Obstruction

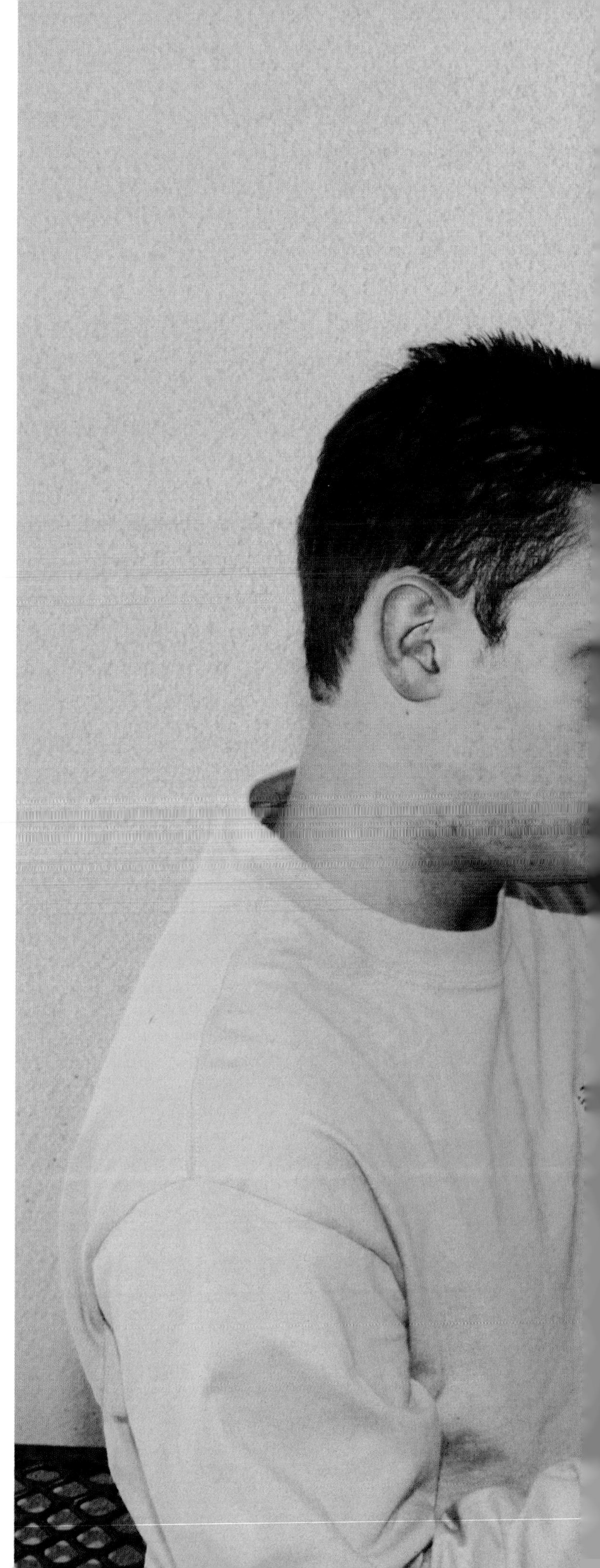

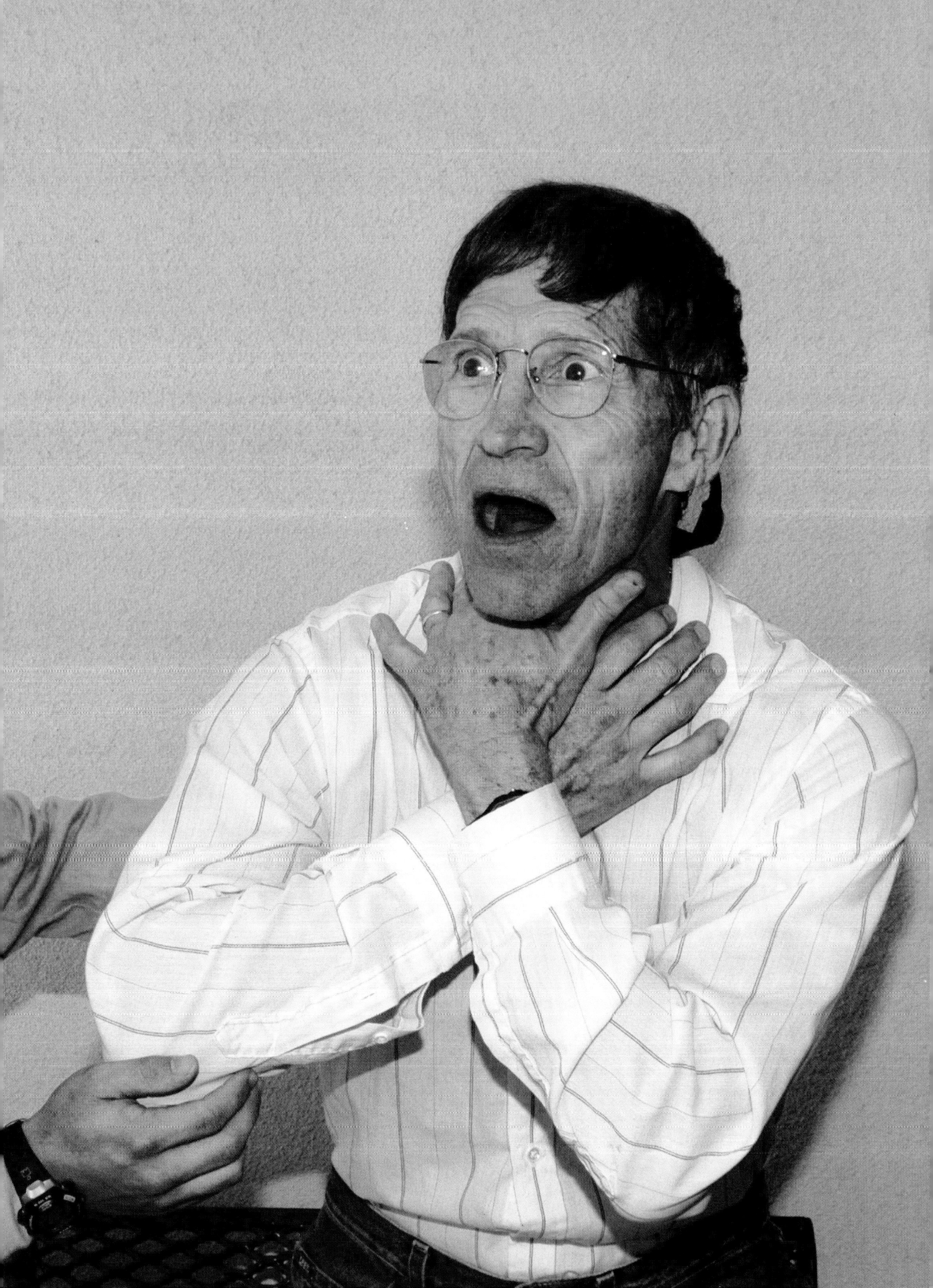

Choking is a common emergency. It is common in infants and children, but more adults than children die from choking each year. Adults can choke for any of the following reasons:

- Swallowing large pieces of poorly chewed food
- Drinking alcohol, which dulls the nerves that aid swallowing
- Wearing dentures, which make it difficult to sense whether food is fully chewed before swallowing
- Eating too fast or eating while laughing

Children are more likely to choke from walking, playing, or running with food or objects in their mouths. They can also choke from swallowing large pieces of poorly chewed food, eating too fast, or eating while laughing.

LEARNING GOALS

In this chapter you will learn about:

- Providing first aid for airway obstruction to conscious victims
- Providing first aid for airway obstruction to unconscious victims

CONSCIOUS VICTIMS

A victim with a blocked airway instinctively clutches at their throat with one or both hands. Recognize this as a universal sign of choking.

Airways can be partially or completely blocked. If a person has a partially blocked airway, they can still breathe (although breathing is difficult). They are still able to cough or make wheezing sounds. They might be able to speak. If they are trying to cough up the object, encourage them to keep coughing.

Whether your victim is an adult, child, or infant, your first step is to let them know you are trained in first aid. Then you must ask them (or their parent or guardian in the case of a child or infant) for their consent to help them.

The specific actions for helping adults, children, and infants are detailed in the following steps.

Adults

If an adult is still breathing, encourage them to keep coughing and trying to bring up the object. If the person continues to cough, but does not cough up the object, they require medical attention. Call for help for this situation.

Use the following series of steps if an adult cannot speak, cough, or breathe due to an airway obstruction:

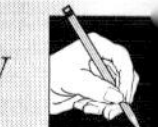

Back Blows

1. Stand to one side and slightly behind the victim.
2. Have the victim bend forward at the waist so that if the object is dislodged it comes out of the mouth rather than falling back into and obstructing the airway.
3. Support the victim with one hand under their chest and with the heel of the other hand deliver up to five sharp back blows between the shoulder blades. Each blow is delivered intending to dislodge the obstruction. They are not intended to be delivered in succession regardless of outcome.
4. If the back blows are not successful and the victim is still conscious use the next method.

Abdominal Thrusts

1. Stand behind the victim.
2. Wrap your arms around the victim's waist.
3. Feel for the victim's navel, and place two fingers of one hand above the navel.
4. Place the fist from your other hand above the two fingers with your thumb facing in.
5. Grasp the fist with the other hand.
6. Perform up to five quick inward and upward abdominal thrusts using your arms.

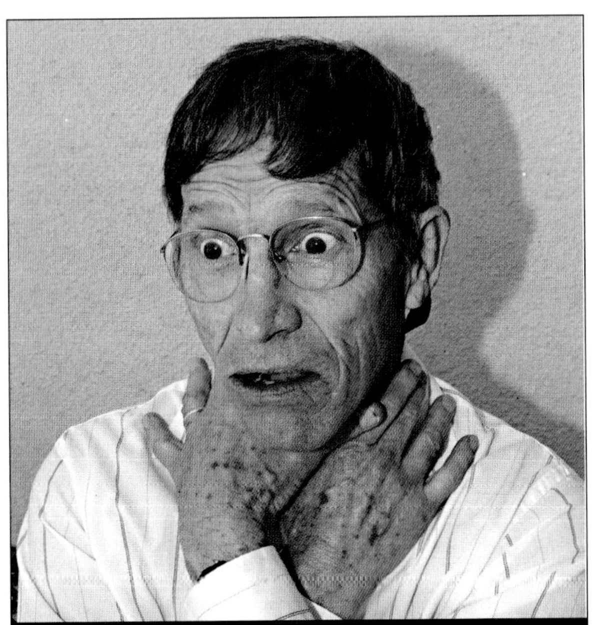

A victim with a blocked airway instinctively clutches at their throat with one or both hands.

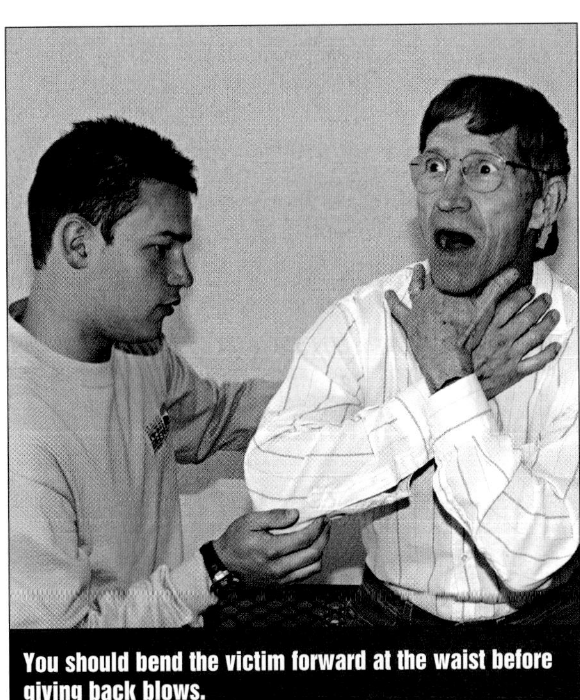

You should bend the victim forward at the waist before giving back blows.

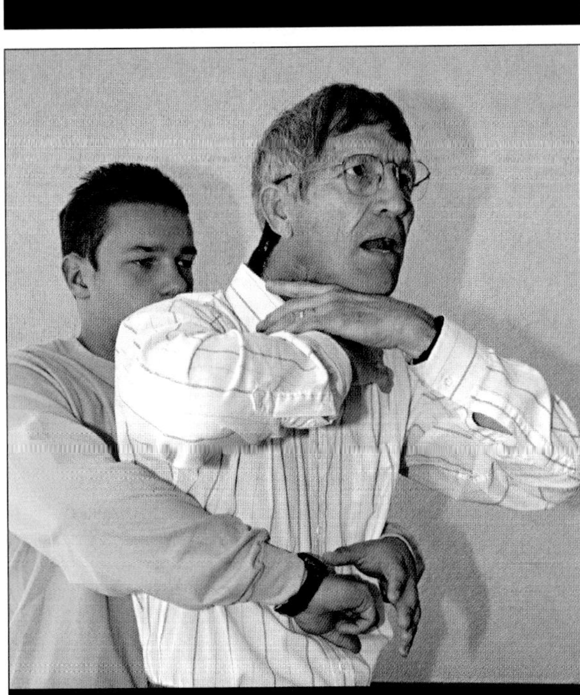

Place your fist against the victim's abdomen with the thumb facing in.

With each thrust you are attempting to dislodge the object with a sudden blast of air. As with back blows, each thrust is intended to dislodge the object.

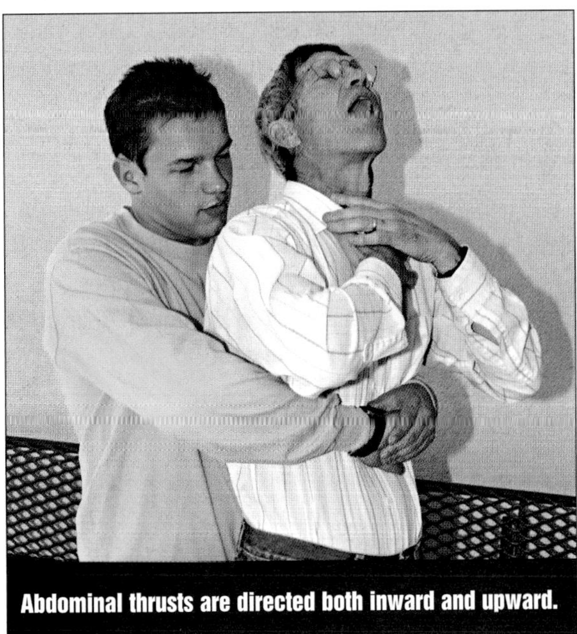

Abdominal thrusts are directed both inward and upward.

7. If the object is not expelled and the person is still conscious, perform five back blows as previously described and continue to alternate methods - back blows followed by abdominal thrusts - until the object is expelled or the person loses consciousness.

8. Lower the person to the ground or floor if they lose consciousness. Activate the emergency response system and begin CPR.

If the person who is choking is obese or pregnant, you must perform chest thrusts instead of abdominal thrusts. Use the following steps to perform chest thrusts:

1. Stand behind the victim.
2. Wrap your arms around the victim's chest.
3. Place a fist from one hand against the center of the victim's breastbone.
4. Grasp the fist with the other hand.
5. Perform up to five quick inward chest thrusts using your arms.
6. If the object is not expelled and the person is still conscious perform five back blows as previously described and continue to alternate methods - back blows followed by abdominal thrusts - until the object is expelled or the person loses consciousness.

Children

If a child is still breathing, encourage them to keep coughing and trying to bring up the object. If the child continues to cough, but does not cough up the object, they require medical attention. Call for help for this situation.

If a child cannot speak, cough, or breathe due to an airway obstruction use the same sequence of steps as for an adult.

Infants

Observe an infant for coughing or crying. If they are actively coughing or crying, watch them closely to see if they expel the object. Use the following steps if the infant is unable to cough or cry:

1. Place the infant, draped over one forearm, face down and with head down. Be sure to support the infant's head and neck with your hand. Support your arm using your thigh.
2. Deliver five back blows to the infant between the shoulder blades. Each blow is delivered intending to dislodge the obstruction. They are not intended to be delivered in succession regardless of outcome.
3. Place your free hand and arm on the infant's head, neck, and torso. In this position, you are sandwiching the infant between your two arms.
4. Turn the infant onto their back on the other forearm. Be sure their head is lower than the trunk of their body.
5. Draw an imaginary line connecting the infant's nipples.
6. Place your index finger, middle finger, and ring finger just below the line.
7. Raise your index finger, leaving the other two fingers on the chest.
8. Deliver five chest thrusts. Do not perform abdominal thrusts on infants.
9. Repeat steps 1 through 8 until the infant expels the object or loses consciousness

UNCONSCIOUS VICTIMS

You might know that a victim is unconscious due to an airway obstruction if they lose consciousness in your presence. However, you might also find someone who is unconscious, and you must determine that the reason is an airway obstruction. Use the following steps to treat an adult, child, or infant who is unconscious due to an airway obstruction.

Adults

Use the following steps if an adult is unconscious, not breathing, and you suspect an airway obstruction:

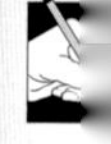

1. Call for help. Activate the emergency response system.
2. Position the victim flat on their back. When positioning a victim, be sure to support their head and neck and keep

it in a straight line with their back. You must position the victim to be lying on a flat, hard surface and on their back.

3. Follow the steps in "Open the Airway" in Chapter 5.
4. Follow the steps in "Check for Breathing" in Chapter 5.
5. Open the victim's mouth and look for an obstruction. If an object is seen you may attempt to remove it with a single finger sweep. Use the finger sweep only if an obstructing object is seen. Using your thumb and forefinger grasp the tongue and lower jaw, open the mouth by lifting and jutting their lower jaw outward, then sweep deeply inside the mouth with a hooked finger to try and remove the object.
6. If your finger sweep is unsuccessful, go to step 7.
7. Give the victim two slow rescue breaths. If the airway is blocked, air will not enter and you will not see the chest rise and fall. Reposition the head to re-open the airway and attempt to ventilate again.
8. If there is no response by the victim, (breathing, coughing, moving) begin chest compressions. (Lifeguards and scuba instructors trained and practiced at locating a carotid pulse should initiate chest compressions even if a pulse is present in a foreign-body-airway-obstructed victim.)
9. Continue with the sequence for CPR for one minute before calling EMS (if this has not already been done).
10. When attempting to deliver subsequent rescue breaths during CPR, look in the victim's mouth for an obstruction.
11. Repeat steps 3 to 10 until you are successful or until help arrives to take over.
12. If you successfully remove or clear the obstruction, continue with "Basic Life Support" as described in Chapter 5.

Children

If a child is unconscious, not breathing, and you suspect an airway obstruction use the same sequence of steps as for an adult. With a child, even if the airway is not blocked you may have to reposition their head several times to correctly open the airway and ventilate.

Infants

Use the following steps if an infant is unconscious, not breathing, and you suspect an airway obstruction:

1. Call for help.
2. Position the victim flat on their back. When positioning a victim, be sure to support their head and neck and keep it in a straight line with their back. You must position the victim to be lying on a flat, hard surface and on their back.
3. Follow the steps in "Open the Airway" in Chapter 5.
4. Follow the steps in "Check for Breathing" in Chapter 5.
5. Give the victim two slow rescue breaths. If the airway is blocked, air will not enter and you will not see the chest rise and fall.
6. Repeat steps 3 to 5 to re-open the airway and ventilate the victim. With an infant, even if the airway is not blocked you may have to reposition their head several times to correctly open the airway and ventilate. If you are still unable to give a successful rescue breath, go to step 7.
7. Place the infant, draped over one forearm, face down and with head down. Be sure to support the infant's head and neck. Support your arm using your thigh.
8. Deliver five back blows to the infant between the shoulder blades.
9. Place your free hand and arm on the infant's head, neck, and torso. In this

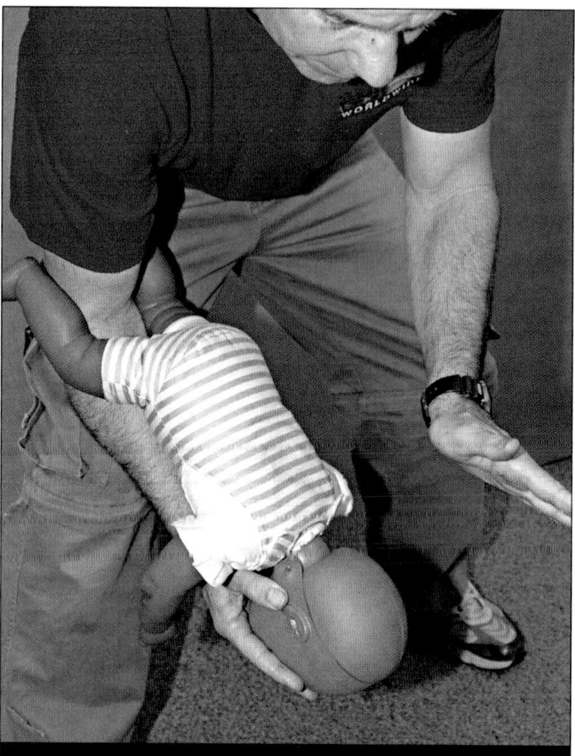

Place the infant, draped over one forearm, face down and with head down. Be sure to support the infant's head and neck with your hand. Support your arm using your thigh.

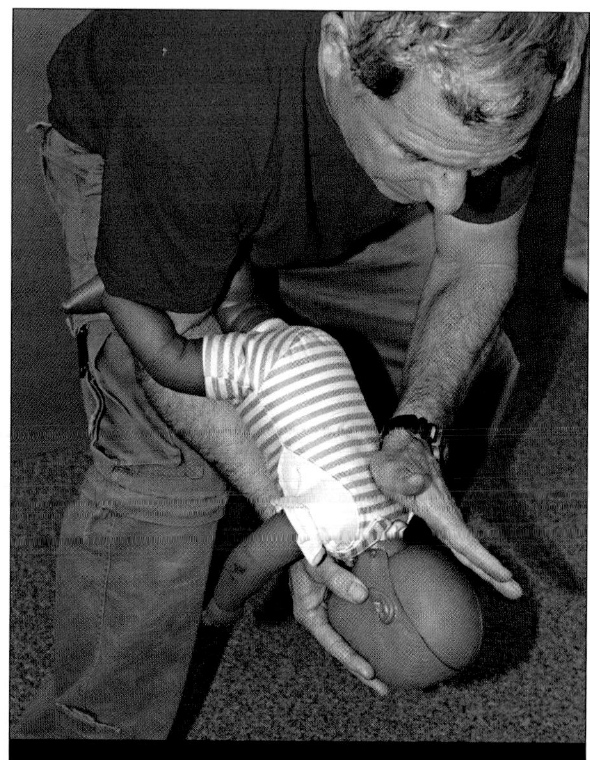

Deliver five back blows to the infant between the shoulder blades.

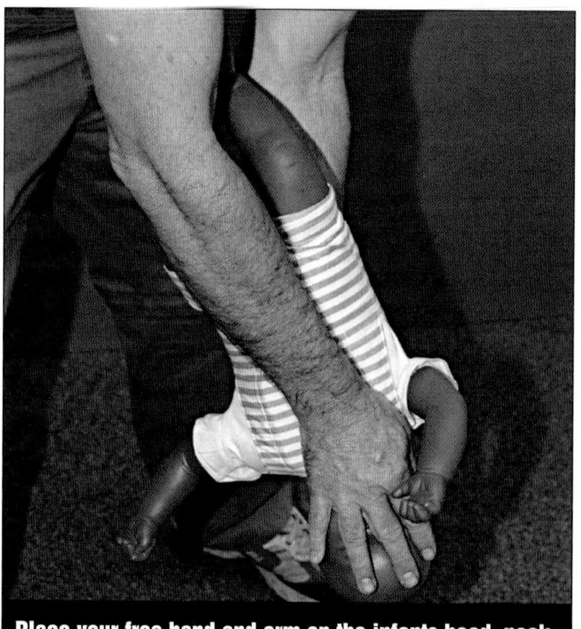

Place your free hand and arm on the infants head, neck and torso and turn the infant onto their back on the other forearm.

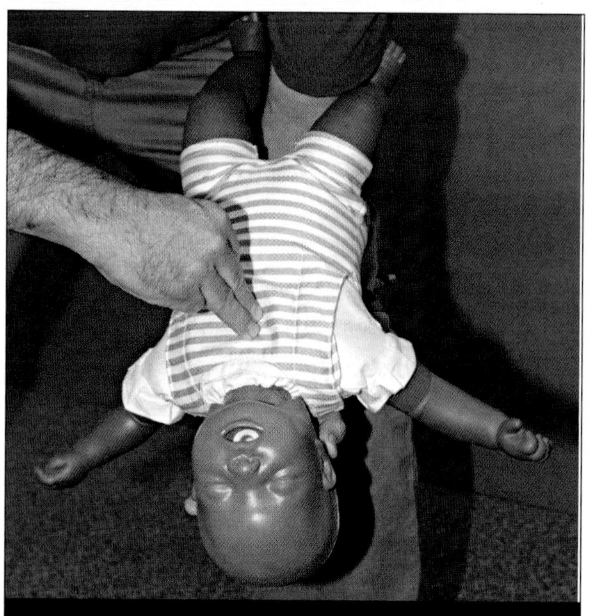

Use your middle and ring fingers in the middle of the infant's breastbone to perform chest thrusts.

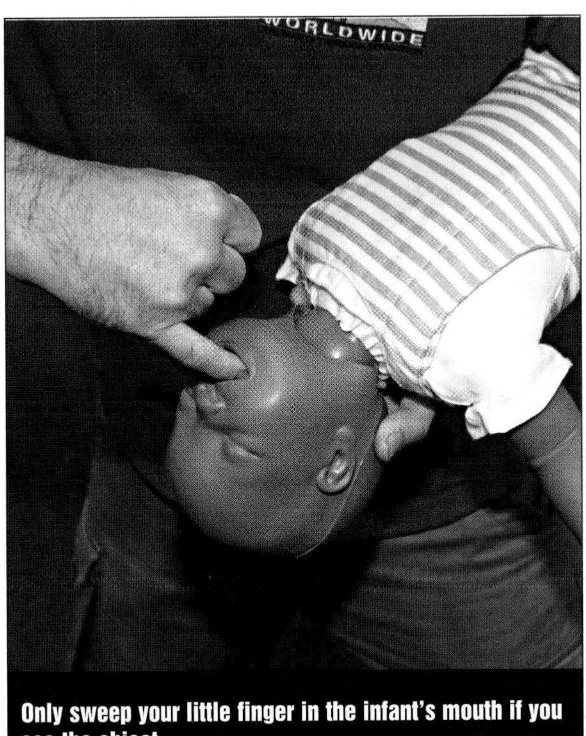

Only sweep your little finger in the infant's mouth if you see the object.

position, you are sandwiching the infant between your two arms.

10. Turn the infant onto their back. Be sure their head is lower than the trunk of their body. Support their head and neck with your hand.
11. Draw an imaginary line connecting the infant's nipples.
12. Place your index finger, middle finger, and ring finger just below the line.
13. Raise your index finger, leaving the other two fingers on the chest.
14. Deliver 5 chest thrusts.
15. Check the mouth for a foreign object. Only sweep your little finger in the infant's mouth if you see the object.
16. Repeat steps 3 to 15 until you are successful or until help arrives to take over.
17. If you successfully remove or clear the obstruction, continue with "Basic Life Support" as described in Chapter 5.

REVIEW QUESTIONS

1. Use the following series of steps if an adult cannot speak, cough, or breathe due to an airway obstruction:

Back Blows

1. ______________________________
____
2. ______________________________
____
3. ______________________________
____
4. ______________________________
____

Abdominal Thrusts

1. ______________________________
____
2. ______________________________
____
3. ______________________________
____
4. ______________________________
____
5. ______________________________
____
6. ______________________________
____
7. ______________________________
____
8. ______________________________
____

2. Use the following steps if an adult is unconscious, not breathing, and you suspect an airway obstruction:

1. ____

2. ____

3. ____

4. ____

5. ____

6. ____

7. ____

8. ____

9. ____

10. ____

11. ____

12. ____

CHAPTER 7

Emergency Oxygen Administration

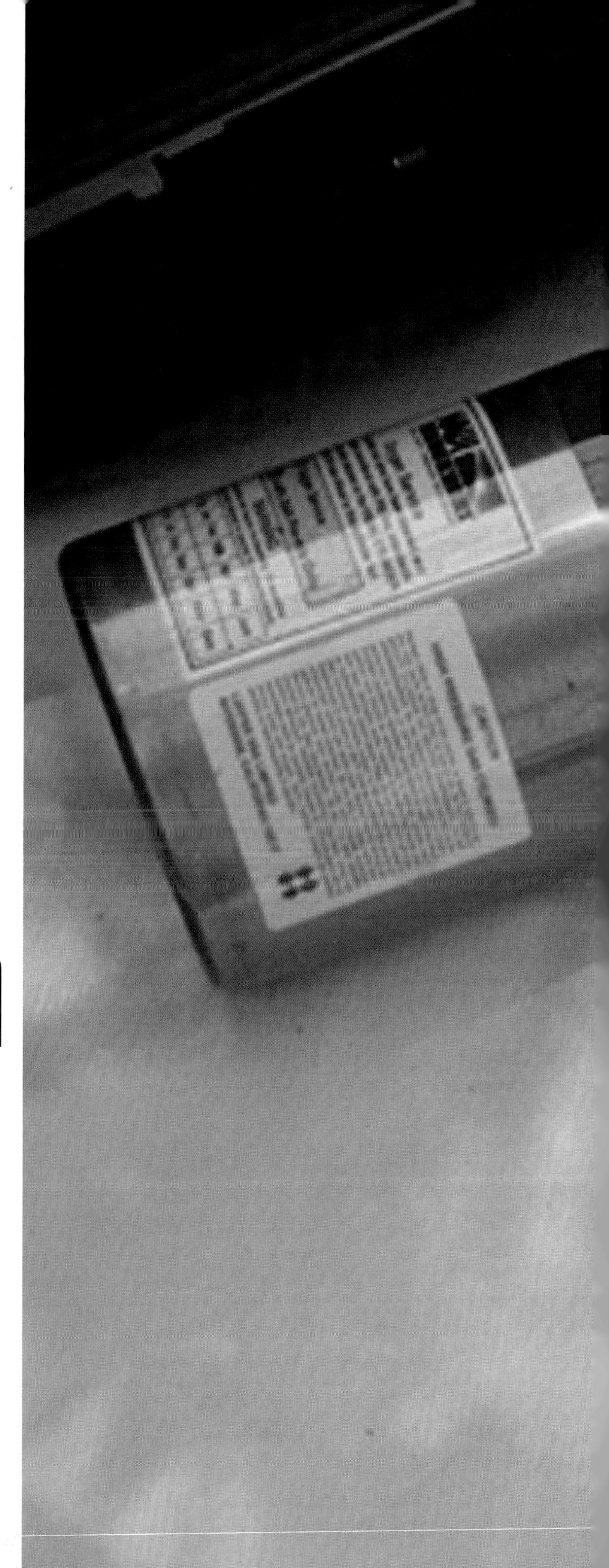

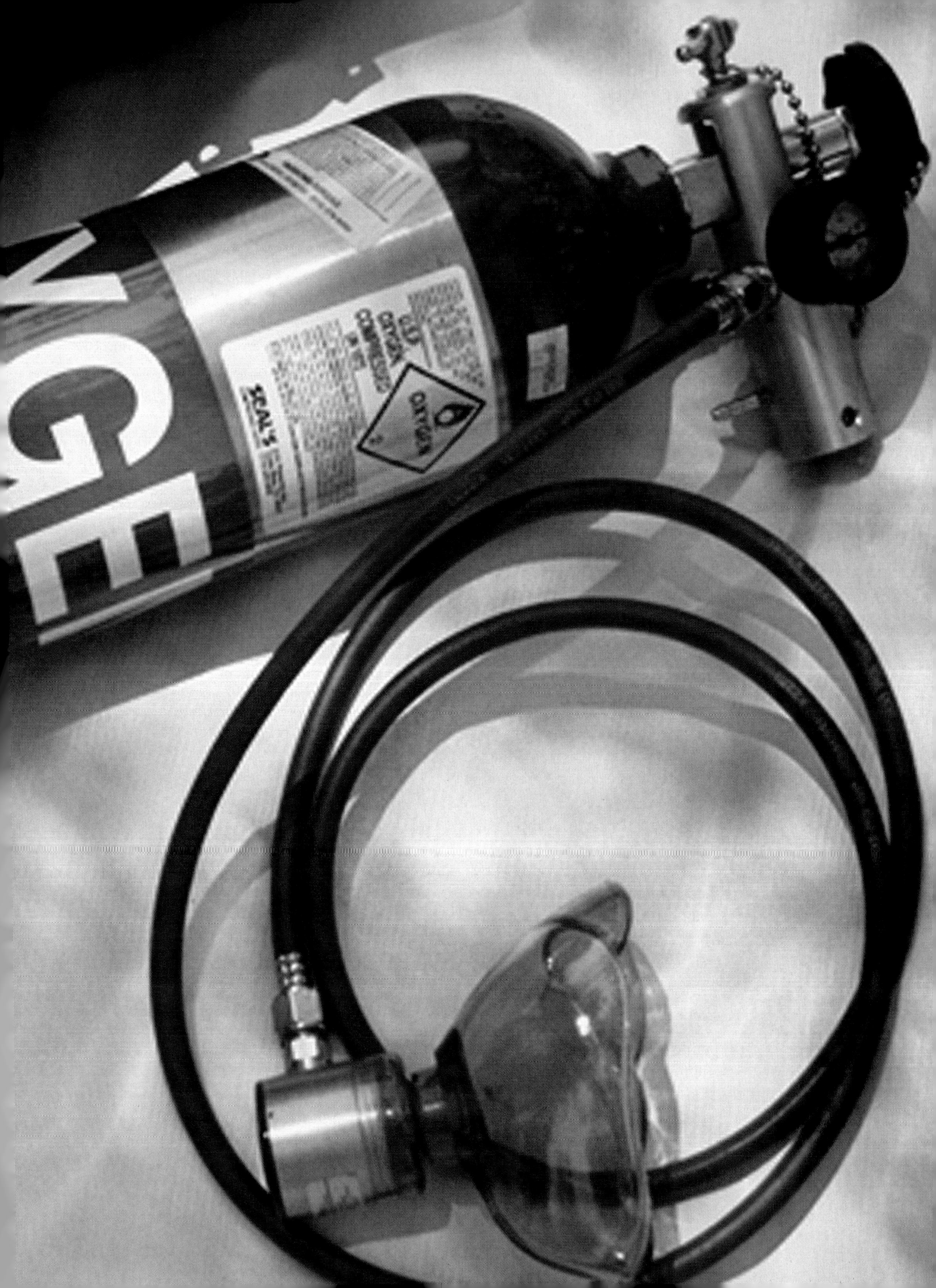

While basic life support intends to maintain a victim's breathing and circulation, adjunct life support improves upon that first aid by adding beneficial support of emergency oxygen and automated external defibrillation (AED). In this section we explore how to best deploy these lifesaving technologies and their proper administration.

LEARNING GOALS

In this chapter you will learn about:

- The value of oxygen in diving maladies and other emergencies
- Precautions associated with handling pure oxygen
- The parts of the emergency oxygen kit
- Administering oxygen to a breathing victim
- Administering oxygen to a non-breathing victim
- Stowing the oxygen kit

VALUE OF OXYGEN IN EMERGENCIES

Oxygen is essential for life. If a person is deprived of oxygen due to illness or injury, permanent damage to the brain and other vital organs can result within a short period of time.

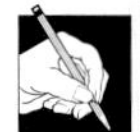

Administering oxygen in the following emergencies can help lessen the permanent damage:

- Decompression sickness
- Arterial gas embolism
- Near-drowning
- Cardiopulmonary emergencies
- Strokes
- Sudden illness

Decompression Sickness

Decompression sickness (DCS) is caused by inert gas (nitrogen) that has been absorbed into a diver's tissues during a dive coming out of solution during and after ascent and forming bubbles in the tissues. When the injured diver breathes 100% oxygen, the nitrogen level in their lungs is reduced towards zero. This creates a high nitrogen pressure gradient in the lungs, bloodstream, and then tissues that enables the ingassed nitrogen to be eliminated at a faster rate. As the dissolved nitrogen in the tissues is eliminated, the offending bubbles start to shrink and then might collapse entirely as nitrogen from the bubbles goes back into solution in the tissues. Properly administering 100% oxygen and keeping the nitrogen pressure gradient as high as possible can result in a significant reduction in bubble size and relief of symptoms.

Another positive effect of administering 100% oxygen in cases of decompression sickness is that it tends to prevent permanence of the inert gas bubbles. The body sees the bubbles as foreign intruders, and tries to encapsulate them to protect the body. The administration of 100% oxygen reduces the size of the bubbles and helps prevent encapsulation.

Bubbles in smaller blood vessels will cause tissues in the surrounding areas to be oxygen-deprived or hypoxic. Over time, this causes the surrounding tissues to swell from fluid retention (edema). Breathing 100% oxygen helps oxygenate these areas and helps prevent the swelling.

Arterial Gas Embolism

In cases of arterial gas embolism (AGE), blood flow to a specific area of the body is interrupted due to a bubble blocking an artery or arteriole. Of special concern are the tissues of the brain and central nervous system, which cannot tolerate oxygen deprivation for more than a few minutes. Administering 100% oxygen will help to oxygenate the tissues surrounding the blockage. This will lessen the risk of permanent damage or death to the tissues affected by the blockage.

Near-Drowning

In the case of a near-drowning, whether there is fluid in the lungs or not (80% have less than a teaspoon of fluid in the lungs) the amount of oxygen delivered to the tissues is compromised (hypoxemia). Breathing 100% oxygen helps to elevate the amount of oxygen in the bloodstream to lessen the effects of hypoxemia.

Cardiopulmonary Emergencies

In respiratory or cardiac distress, the body has a limited ability to circulate oxygen-rich blood to the tissues. People in respiratory or cardiac distress have a critical need for emergency oxygen to help prevent damage to the brain and heart. Emergency oxygen should be administered during cardiac or respiratory emergencies as soon as it is available.

Sudden Illness

You should administer oxygen to anyone experiencing a sudden illness, whether they are responsive or unresponsive. It will enhance the likelihood of a better outcome for the person.

OXYGEN PRECAUTIONS

Heat, fuel, and oxygen, sometimes called the "fire triangle," are necessary to have a fire. In the presence of pure oxygen, plus heat and fuel, a fire will be much larger and more violent than when burning in ordinary air.

When you are handling any pure oxygen or high-percentage oxygen gas mixture, you must reduce the risk of a fire. Work in a well-ventilated area. Be sure that all hazards due to fuel (oil deposits, diesel fuel or gasoline, and any other hydrocarbons) are not near the oxygen cylinder. Try not to position the oxygen cylinder in the sun or close to a hot engine. Open the oxygen cylinder valve slowly when you need to use oxygen.

Some safety precautions to follow with oxygen cylinders and oxygen units are:

- Do not allow any grease or oil to come in contact with the oxygen cylinder, regulator, or the oxygen kit.
- Do not expose oxygen cylinders to temperatures over 125° Fahrenheit (52° Celsius) when in storage.

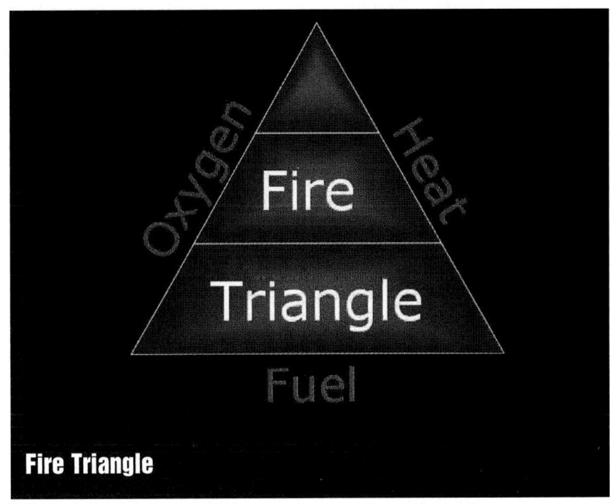

Fire Triangle

- Do not allow smoking or any open flames near an oxygen cylinder or kit.
- Provide adequate ventilation when using oxygen.
- Use only the equipment (cylinders, regulators, gauges, and valves) intended for use with oxygen. Do not modify other equipment to use it with oxygen.
- Inspect the condition of the valves and washers to be sure they are compatible to use with oxygen.
- Do not touch the surface of the oxygen cylinder valve opening or regulator orifice with your fingers as the body oil residue left on their surfaces could ignite when the oxygen valve is opened.

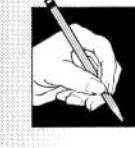

- Open the cylinder valve slowly and only enough to allow oxygen to flow unrestricted. There is no need to open the valve all the way. One full turn is sufficient.
- Keep the valve closed, with the system assembled but purged when oxygen is not in use.
- Do not store oxygen cylinders empty.
- Always secure oxygen cylinders so they cannot fall or roll, that is, lay them down when administering oxygen first aid.

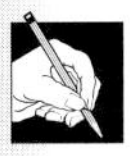

- Carry an oxygen cylinder with two hands and avoid holding it by the valve or regulator.

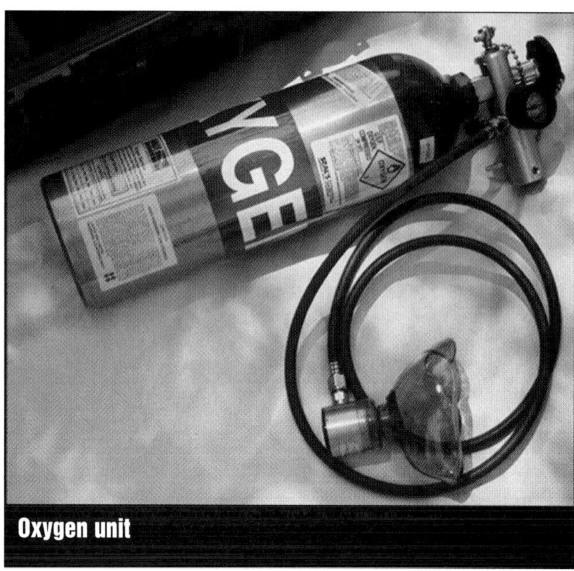

Oxygen unit

- Have the oxygen cylinder hydrostatically tested when testing is due (every five years in the United States).

OXYGEN UNIT DESCRIPTION

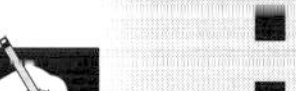

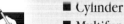

An oxygen unit consists of the following items:

- Cylinder
- Multifunction regulator
- Demand inhalator valve
- Masks

Medical oxygen applications use an adjustable free-flow regulator and any of several constant-flow masks and nasal canula to deliver the oxygen to the patient. Medical oxygen units are usually used where additional oxygen cylinders are readily available. For diving maladies, a demand valve system is preferred because:

- The cylinder will last longer because oxygen flows only when the patient inhales.
- The demand inhalator valve is able to deliver 100% oxygen to the patient with each inhalation.

Oxygen units are stored with the regulator attached to the valve, the intermediate pressure hose attached to the regulator, the demand inhalator valve attached to the intermediate pressure hose, and the oxygen turned off and the system

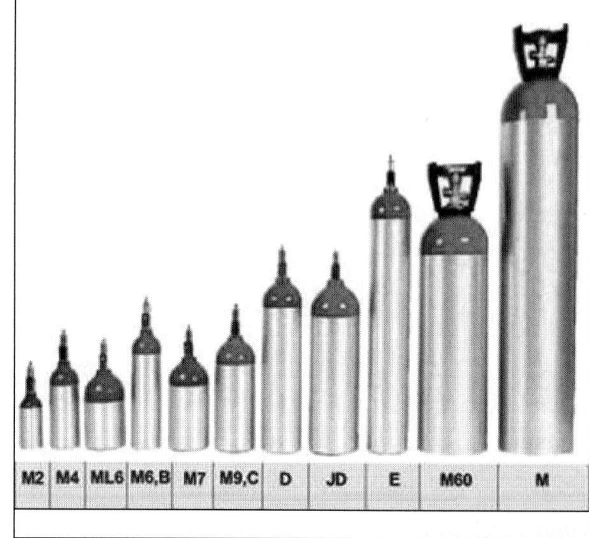

Oxygen cylinders come in different sizes from small portable cylinders to large, non-portable.

purged. The unit is always ready to be used when needed.

Cylinders

Oxygen cylinders come in different sizes from small portable cylinders to large, non-portable cylinders. The size you need depends on the proximity of medical services to your site. Oxygen cylinders can be made from aluminum or steel and are subject to periodic hydrostatic testing.

Oxygen cylinders are color-coded for easy identification. In the United States, they are green (steel) or silver with a green shoulder (aluminum). In Canada and Europe, they are white. In Australia, New Zealand, the United Kingdom, and other countries, they are black with a white shoulder. Some standard cylinder sizes for oxygen first aid are:

- The E cylinder, which holds 24 cubic feet (680 liters) of compressed gas.
- The Jumbo D cylinder, which holds 22 cubic feet (623 liters) of compressed gas.
- The D cylinder, which holds 15 cubic feet (425 liters) of compressed gas.
- The C cylinder, which holds 9 cubic feet

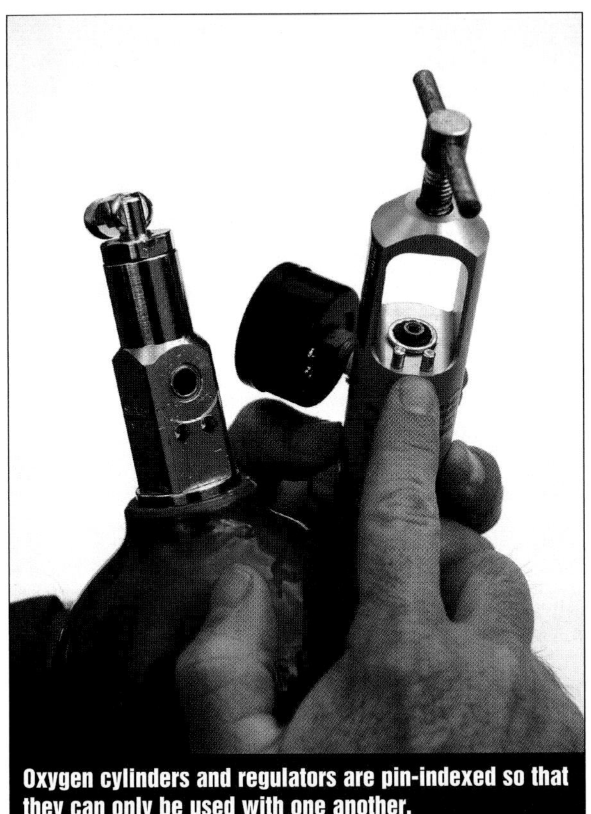

Oxygen cylinders and regulators are pin-indexed so that they can only be used with one another.

(255 liters) of compressed gas.

Oxygen cylinders also have specific valves that only accept oxygen regulators. The pin-indexed valve (Compressed Gas Association [CGA] 870 medical oxygen valve) has two holes that engage pins located on the oxygen regulator. The pins are placed in a specific orientation to prevent the regulator from being used on a cylinder that does not contain oxygen.

The threaded gas-outlet valve (CGA 540 medical oxygen valve or bull-nose valve), used on large cylinders, will only accept a regulator intended for medical oxygen use. Your instructor will let you know which type of regulator is used in your region.

Multifunction Regulator

The multifunction regulator reduces the cylinder pressure to a lower working pressure, just like the first stage of a scuba regulator reduces cylinder pressure to an intermediate pressure. As the name implies, it can be used either as a free-flow system first stage or as a demand-valve system first stage. The multifunction regulator has the following parts:

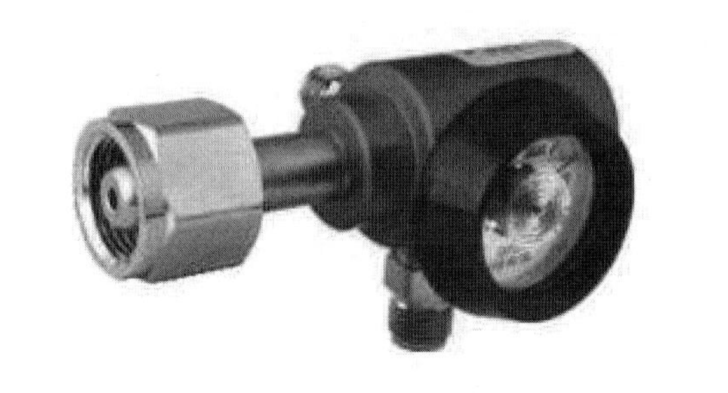

CGA 540 medical oxygen valve or bull-nose valve

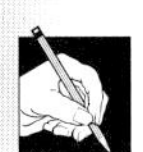

- Threaded outlets that are used with demand inhalator valves. The regulator might have one or two of these outlets. The outlets have a safety valve that closes if a demand inhalator valve hose is not attached.
- A constant flow outlet. The constant flow outlet can be adjusted to deliver up to 25 liters per minute to a constant-flow facemask device.
- A constant flow meter which regulates and indicates the flow rate to the constant-flow facemask.
- A pressure gauge indicating the pressure in the oxygen cylinder.

The multifunction regulator is attached to the oxygen cylinder through either a yoke configuration like some scuba regulator first stages, or a threaded inlet valve.

Demand Inhalator Valve

The demand valve is like the second stage of a scuba regulator. It is attached to the multifunction regulator by an intermediate-pressure hose that is threaded at both ends. One end of the hose threads onto the threaded outlet on the multifunc-

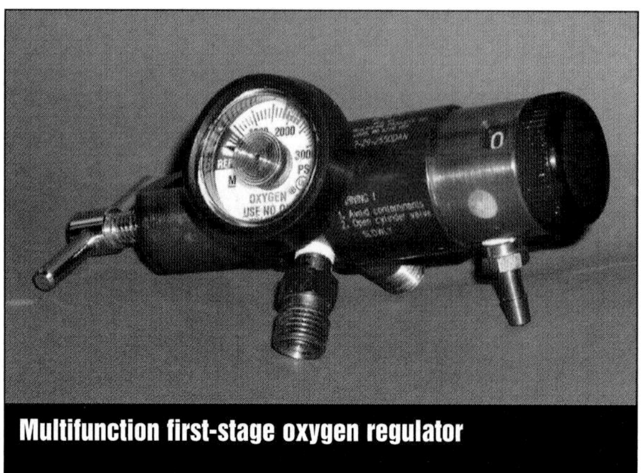
Multifunction first-stage oxygen regulator

tion regulator at the cylinder and the other end threads onto the demand valve at the face mask. Unlike a scuba regulator intermediate-pressure hose, the two threaded ends are interchangeable.

The demand valve will only provide oxygen when the user breathes in. This ensures that the oxygen supply will last longer than a constant flow system. Different types of masks that fit over both the user's mouth and nose can be attached to the demand valve.

Masks

Oxygen masks and their tubing are manufactured from oxygen-safe material.

The clear oronasal mask attaches directly to the demand valve. On the user, it fits over both the nose and mouth. This oronasal mask provides a good seal for most faces. This mask provides close to 100% oxygen (as long as a proper seal is maintained) and enables the oxygen supply to last longer than if a constant-flow system is being used.

An oronasal/barrier rescue-breathing mask (pocket mask) can also be attached to the demand valve at the one-way valve and would be used if a good seal cannot be obtained with the standard oronasal mask. The pocket mask also covers the nose and mouth and can be held in place with an adjustable elastic band.

The pocket mask can also be used with the constant flow outlet. In this case, clear plastic

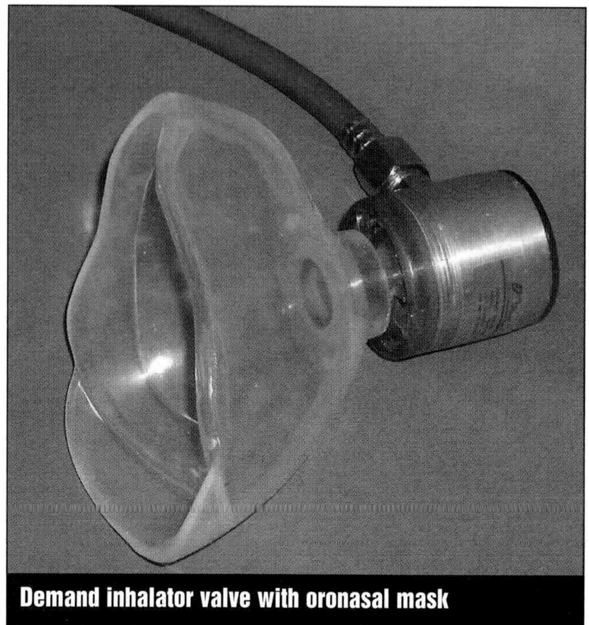
Demand inhalator valve with oronasal mask

tubing is attached from the regulator's constant flow outlet to the oxygen inlet on the pocket mask. The pocket mask can also be used for a non-breathing victim. Oxygen is supplied at constant flow through the oxygen inlet, while a rescuer breathes for the victim through the one-way valve.

The non-rebreather mask is used with the constant flow outlet. Clear plastic tubing attaches to the constant flow outlet and to the oxygen inlet on the non-rebreather mask. The non-rebreather mask also covers the nose and mouth and can be held in place with an adjustable elastic band. The mask has a reservoir bag attached to it, and three non-return (one-way) valves. Two of the non-return valves are located on either side of the mask, and the third non-return valve is located between the reservoir bag and the mask. Oxygen flows into the reservoir bag. When the user inhales, oxygen is drawn from the reservoir bag into the mask. When the user exhales, the expired air vents to outside the mask through the non-return valves on either side of the mask. As the user exhales, the reservoir bag refills with oxygen for the next breath. The non-rebreather mask will deliver up to 90% pure oxygen with a proper fit. However, 65 to 75% delivery is common.

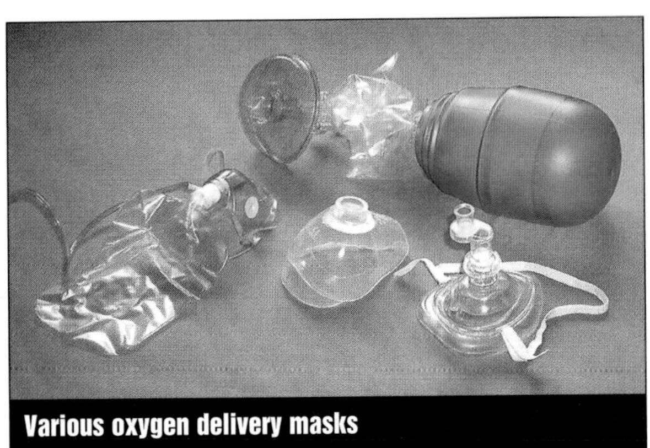

Various oxygen delivery masks

The bag-valve-mask also covers the nose and mouth and consists of a clear plastic mask, a self-filling bag, and an oxygen reservoir with an oxygen inlet. This mask is used for non breathing victims or for victims with weak respirations. The rescuer ventilates the victim by squeezing the self-filling bag. This mask can deliver oxygen in concentrations up to 90%, but it is difficult to use effectively. The rescuer must be well trained in its use and practice frequently to maintain their skills. The most common problem is maintaining a good seal between the mask and the victim's face.

ADMINISTERING EMERGENCY OXYGEN

When you are administering emergency oxygen, your victim will either be breathing or not breathing. The steps for each type of victim are slightly different and are outlined in the following sections. Your first steps, in either case, are to assess the scene as follows:

1. If you are administering oxygen in a diving emergency, perform the following steps:
   a. Ensure that all the scuba gear is secure so that it will not roll or fall.
   b. Recall all the divers.
2. Check to be sure that the ventilation is adequate for oxygen to be administered.
3. Check to be sure that all smoking materials have been extinguished.
4. Use barrier devices such as gloves and mouth-to-mask devices.

BREATHING VICTIMS

Use the following steps when you have a breathing, conscious victim who needs emergency oxygen and you are using the demand inhalator valve with either an oronasal mask or pocket mask:

1. Ask the victim if they need assistance.
2. Identify yourself and let them know you are trained to administer oxygen.
3. Tell them that oxygen might help them and ask if they want to breathe it. 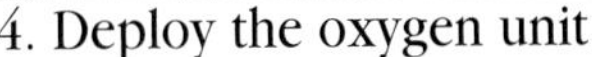 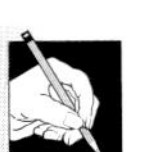
4. Deploy the oxygen unit:
   a. Open the cylinder valve with one complete turn. Open the valve slowly. Be sure the pressure gauge is pointed away from you, the victim and any bystanders.
   b. Check the cylinder pressure.
   c. Check that there are no leaks in the system. If there are leaks, shut the unit down and fix the leaks.
   d. Check that the constant flow setting is at zero (0) or the off position.
   e. Inhale a breath of oxygen through the demand inhalator valve's mask. This will assure that the system is functioning properly and will also demonstrate to the victim that it is working. Exhale after you have removed the mask from your face.
5. Place the mask over the victim's mouth and nose.
6. Tell the victim to breathe normally from the mask.
7. Comfort the victim.
8. Ask the victim to hold the mask to their face to help maintain an effective seal.
9. Monitor the victim and the pressure gauge:
   a. Listen for the demand inhalator valve to open.
   b. Look for the mask to fog from exhaled breath.

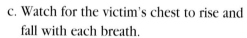

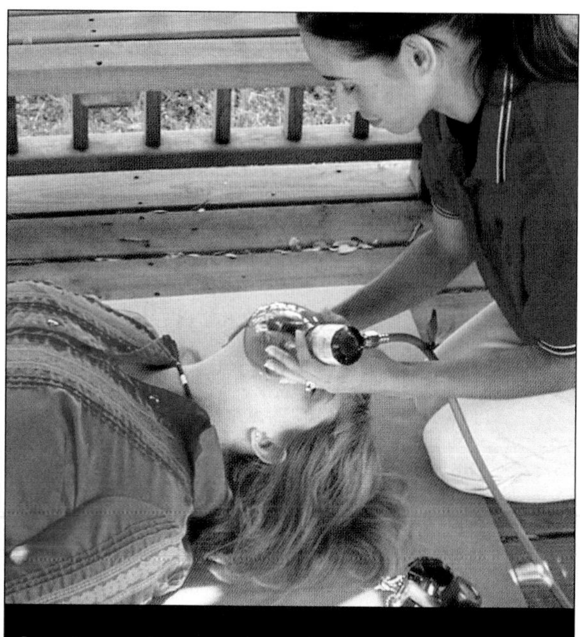
Conscious victim using demand valve and oronasal mask

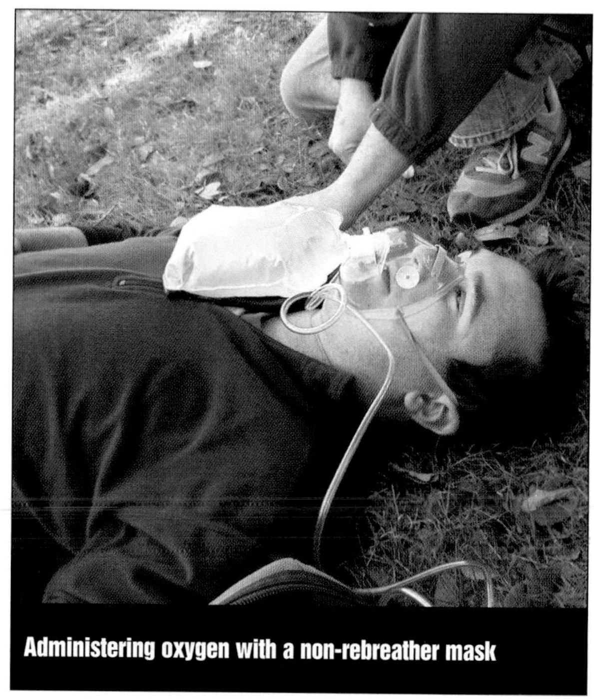
Administering oxygen with a non-rebreather mask

c. Watch for the victim's chest to rise and fall with each breath.

d. Check to be sure the cylinder is not running out of oxygen.

10. Call for help.
11. If you are administering oxygen in a diving emergency, perform the following steps:
    a. Call Divers Alert Network (DAN). They will begin the communication process between you, the nearest medical facility, the nearest recompression chamber, the recompression chamber personnel, and any necessary evacuation personnel.
    b. Once you have begun to administer oxygen, use it all. Do not try to stretch out the supply or conserve oxygen by shutting down the unit for "air breaks" - even if symptoms are relieved.
    c. Transport the victim to the nearest medical facility with subsequent transport to a hyperbaric chamber.

Use the following steps when you have a breathing, conscious victim who needs emergency oxygen and you are using the constant flow oxygen with a non-rebreather mask:

1. Ask the victim if they need assistance.
2. Identify yourself and let them know you are trained to administer oxygen.
3. Tell them that oxygen might help them and ask if they want to breathe it.
4. Deploy the oxygen unit:
   a. Attach the oxygen tubing to the constant flow outlet.
   b. If it is not already attached to the mask, attach the other end of the oxygen tubing to the oxygen inlet on the non-rebreather mask.
   c. Open the cylinder valve with one complete turn. Open the valve slowly. Be sure the pressure gauge is pointed away from you, the victim, and any bystanders.
   d. Check the cylinder pressure.
   e. Check that there are no leaks in the system. If there are leaks, shut the unit down and fix the leaks.
   f. Set the constant flow setting to 15 liters per minute.

g. Hold your finger over the non-return valve to the reservoir bag to inflate the bag with oxygen.

5. Place the mask over the victim's mouth and nose.
6. Adjust the elastic band around the victim's head to hold the mask in place.
7. Squeeze the metal clip over the victim's nose to help prevent leakage of oxygen from the mask.
8. Tell the victim to breathe normally from the mask.
9. If the victim is breathing heavily and completely deflating the reservoir bag with each breath, increase the oxygen flow rate.
10. Comfort the victim.
11. Ask the victim to hold the mask to their face to help maintain an effective seal.
12. Monitor the victim and the pressure gauge:
    a Look for the mask to fog from exhaled breath.
    b Watch for the victim's chest to rise and fall with each breath.
    c Check to be sure the cylinder is not running out of oxygen.
13. Call for help.
14. If you are administering oxygen in a diving emergency, perform the following steps:
    a. Call Divers Alert Network (DAN). They will begin the communication process between you, the nearest medical facility, the nearest recompression chamber, the recompression chamber personnel, and any necessary evacuation personnel.
    b. Once you have begun to administer oxygen, use it all. Do not try to stretch out the supply or conserve oxygen by shutting down the unit for "air breaks" - even if symptoms are relieved.
    c. Transport the victim to the nearest medical facility with subsequent transport to a hyperbaric chamber.

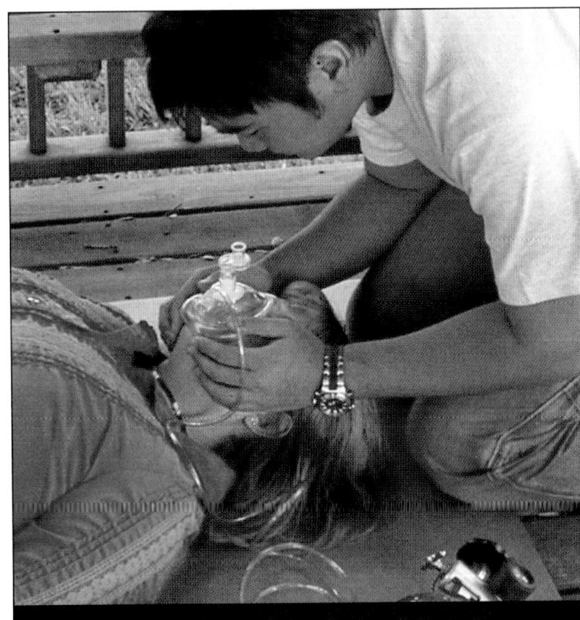

Performing rescue breathing with a pocket mask and supplemental oxygen

NON-BREATHING VICTIMS

Use the following steps when you have a non-breathing victim who needs emergency oxygen and you are using the pocket mask and constant-flow oxygen:

1. Check the victim for responsiveness.
2. Call for help.
3. Check for airway and breathing. See Section 3, Chapter 5 for the specific steps.
4. Deploy the oxygen unit: (Have someone administer rescue breathing while you are deploying the unit.)
    a. Attach the oxygen tubing to the constant flow outlet.
    b. Attach the other end of the oxygen tubing to the oxygen inlet on the pocket mask.
    c. Open the cylinder valve with one complete turn. Open the valve slowly. Be sure the pressure gauge is pointed away from you, the victim, and any bystanders.
    d. Check the cylinder pressure.
    e. Check that there are no leaks in the system. If there are leaks, shut the unit down and fix the leaks.

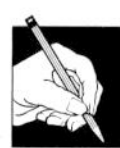

f. Set the constant flow setting to 15 liters per minute.

5. Place the mask over the victim's mouth and nose.
6. Recheck for airway, breathing, and circulation.
7. Using the base of the thumbs and fingers to hold the mask firmly in place and make a seal, start rescue breathing through the one-way valve.
8. If you are administering oxygen in a diving emergency, perform the following steps:
   a. Call Divers Alert Network (DAN). They will begin the communication process between you, the nearest medical facility, the nearest recompression chamber, the recompression chamber personnel, and any necessary evacuation personnel.
   b. Once you have begun to administer oxygen, use it all. Do not try to stretch out the supply or conserve oxygen by shutting down the unit for "air breaks" - even if symptoms are relieved.
   c. Transport the victim to the nearest medical facility with subsequent transport to a hyperbaric chamber.

STOWING THE OXYGEN UNIT

Use the following steps to store the oxygen unit after it has been used:

1. Turn off the oxygen unit.
2. Depressurize the lines by turning the constant-flow control to fully on until no more oxygen flows through the lines.
3. Take the regulator off the oxygen cylinder.
4. Take the cylinder to a facility providing medical grade oxygen to be refilled.
5. When the filled cylinder is returned, or if another is available, replace the oxygen regulator on the cylinder.

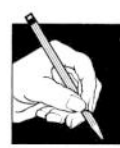

6. Clean the oronasal mask or pocket mask using a mild (10%) bleach and water solution. Soak the mask in the solution, rinse it well with fresh water, and let it dry. Replace a used non-rebreather mask.
7. Ensure that the intermediate pressure hose is securely screwed onto the regulator and the demand inhalator valve.
8. Ensure that the constant flow indicator is set to zero (0).
9. Secure the unit in its protective case.
10. Store the unit in an easily accessible place.

REVIEW QUESTIONS

1. Administering oxygen in the following emergencies can help lessen the permanent damage - list 4 of the 6 examples from the text. ____________________

____

____

2. Do not allow any ____________ to come in contact with the oxygen cylinder, regulator, or the oxygen kit.

3. Do not touch the surface of the oxygen cylinder valve opening or regulator orifice with ____________________ could ignite when the oxygen valve is opened.

4. Always secure oxygen cylinders so they cannot fall or roll, that is, ____________ when administering oxygen first aid.

5. An oxygen unit consists of the following items: ____________________

____________________.

6. Oxygen cylinders are ____________________ for easy identification.

7. A multifunction regulator can be used either as a ____________ or as a ____

____________________.

8. When administering emergency oxygen to a conscious victim you must ____________

____________________.

9. When administering emergency oxygen to a unconscious victim set the constant flow setting to

____________________.

10. When storing the oxygen unit after it has been used, clean the oronasal mask or pocket mask using ____________________.

CHAPTER 8

Automated External Defibrillator

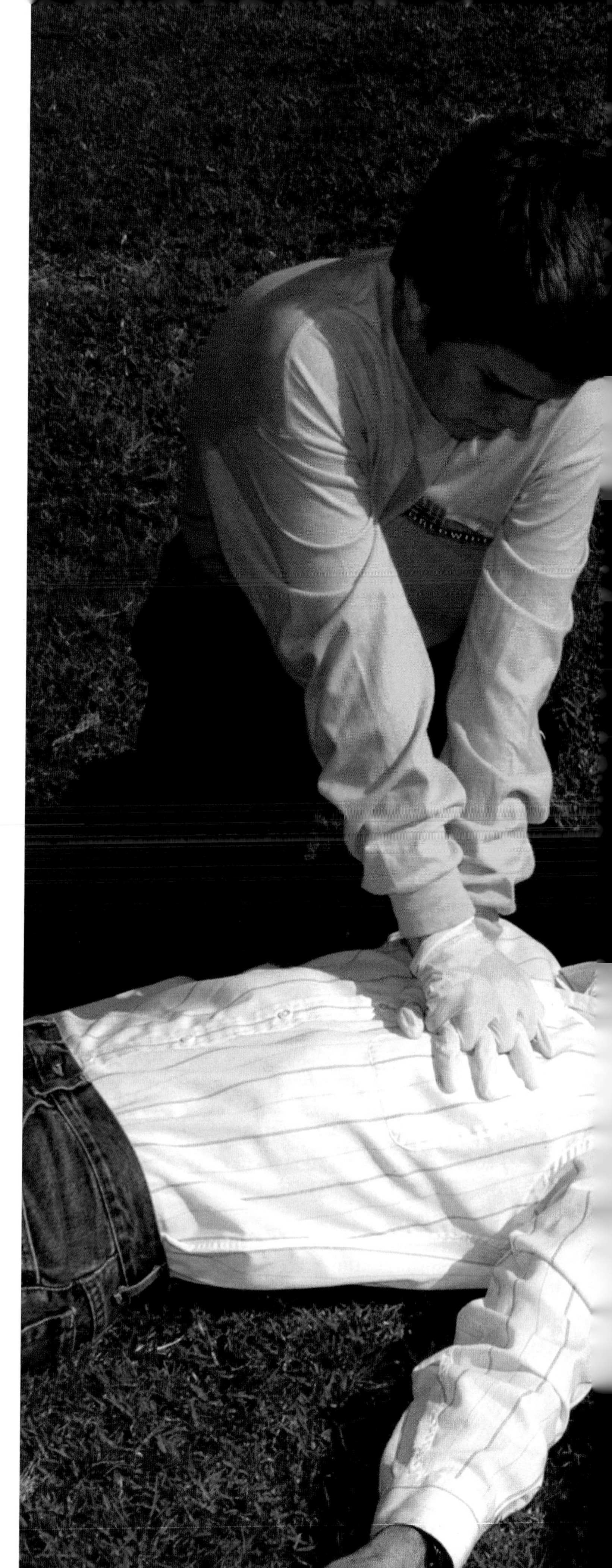

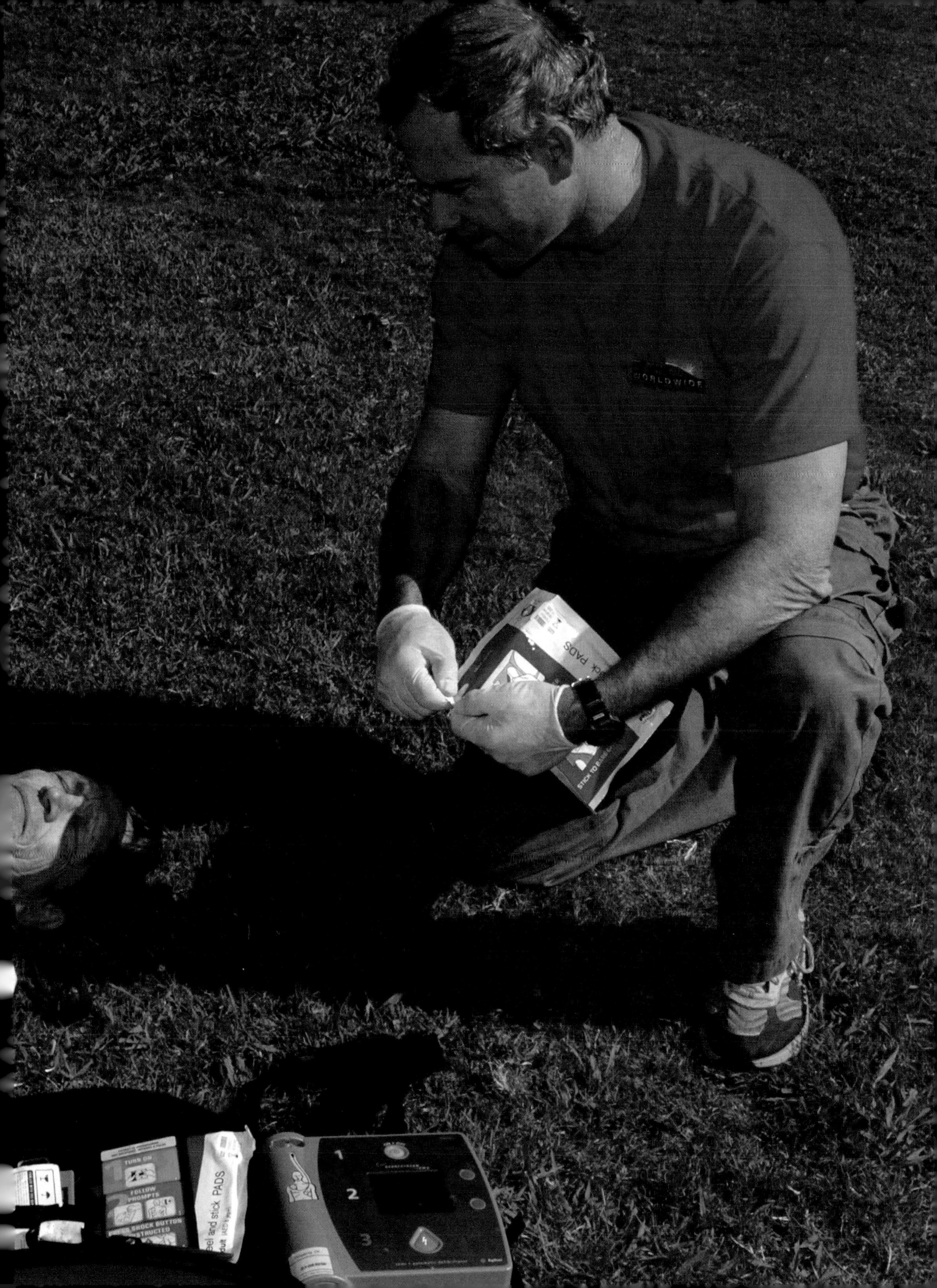
WORLDWIDE
TURN ON
FOLLOW PROMPTS
PADS
1
2
3

No agency collects statistical data on the effectiveness of AED or CPR on a national level although many studies have been conducted in specific communities. These studies have all demonstrated the benefit of early CPR and defibrillation within three to five minutes of a witnessed sudden cardiac arrest. In cities, e.g., Seattle Washington, USA, where advanced care response is rapid and a high proportion of citizens are trained in CPR and the use of AED, survival rates of sudden cardiac arrest victims are as high as thirty percent. Whereas in communities, e.g., New York City, USA, where advanced care response is longer and few victims receive bystander CPR and defibrillation survival of sudden cardiac arrest victims averages only one to two percent.

LEARNING GOALS

In this chapter you will learn about:

- The value of using an automated external defibrillator (AED)
- Preparing the AED for use
- Positioning the AED pads on a victim's chest
- Safely operating the AED

Anyone who has been trained in the use of AEDs can assist in a cardiac emergency.

VALUE OF AUTOMATED EXTERNAL DEFIBRILLATORS

The AED is an external device that reads the victim's heart rhythm pattern and determines if an electrical shock needs to be administered to restart a heart that is twitching or contracting irregularly rather than beating rhythmically. When the rescuer presses a shock button, the AED delivers the electrical shock. The AED should be used within five to six minutes of sudden cardiac arrest (SCA). Survival of the victim has increased to as high as 49% when rescuers administer CPR and a shock from an AED within three to five minutes of SCA.

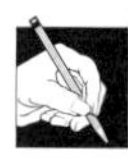

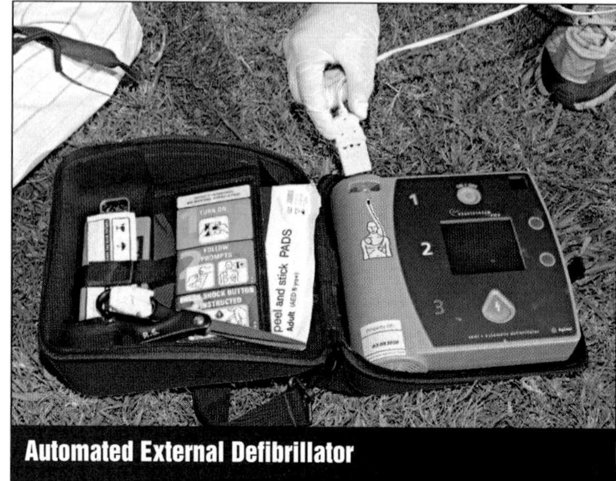

Automated External Defibrillator

Because of this time constraint, AEDs are becoming more common in public places. Airports, airplanes, stadiums, casinos, shopping malls, health clubs, golf courses, and charter dive boats are some of the public places in which you will find AEDs. The facilities purchase these devices under the Public Access Defibrillation (PAD) program. These programs are overseen by a physician and have the following requirements:

- The program must be overseen by a physician.
- The physician must write a prescription to the facility for the purchase of the AED.
- The AED can only be used by individuals with proper training and certification in accordance with local laws.

The laws and regulations affecting the use of AEDs vary widely. Communities or facilities that implement AED programs must check with their local Emergency Medical Services agencies for the laws and regulations in their area.

In the United States, one company, Philips Medical Systems of Andover, Massachusetts, has received marketing clearance from the United States Food and Drug Administration to sell their HeartStart Home Defibrillator without the need for a prescription from a physician. This device can be used safely and effectively by lay people based on written instructions and the device itself.

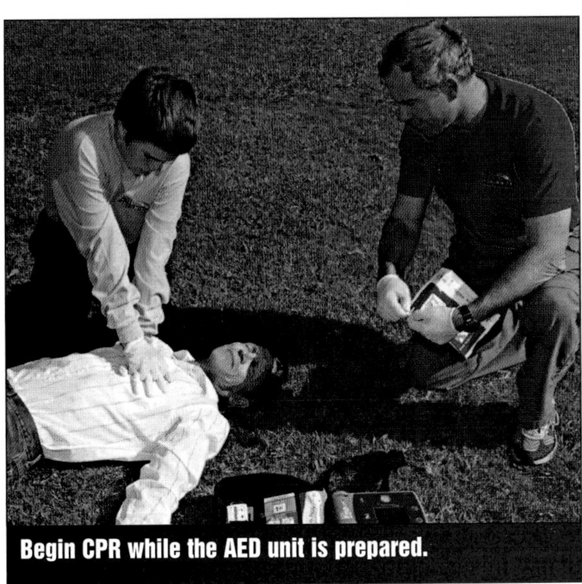
Begin CPR while the AED unit is prepared.

USING THE AUTOMATED EXTERNAL DEFIBRILLATOR FOR ADULTS

Standard AEDs are calibrated for adults and children over eight years old. Some models are equipped with pediatric sized electrode pads and have child modes for use on victims as young as one year. However, in the event these options are not available use the standard AED on children one to eight. It is not recommended on victims less than one year old. They are always used in conjunction with cardiopulmonary resuscitation (CPR). Use the following steps if you encounter a person who has had a sudden cardiac arrest:

1. Call for help.
2. Have a bystander retrieve the AED from its storage unit while you begin CPR.
3. In the event that you are alone and you have witnessed the cardiac arrest, leave the victim to activate the emergency response system and retrieve the AED from its storage unit.
4. In the event that you are alone and did not witness the cardiac arrest or you know it is an asphyxial arrest (for example, a drowning victim) provide 5 cycles of CPR (about 2 minutes) before leaving the victim to activate the emergency response system and retrieve the AED.
5. Position the AED near the victim's left ear.
6. Position yourself on the right side of the victim.
7. Check the victim's airway.
8. Check for breathing.
9. Start CPR if no breathing is present.
10. Power on the AED.
11. Expose the skin of the victim's chest.
12. Attach the electrode pads to the victim's chest. Use the following guidelines when attaching the electrodes:

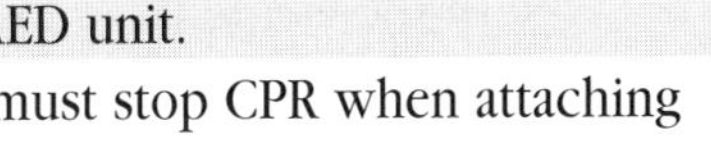

a. The correct placement of the pads is illustrated either on the pads or on the AED unit.

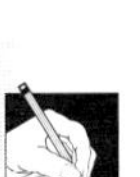

b. You must stop CPR when attaching the pads.

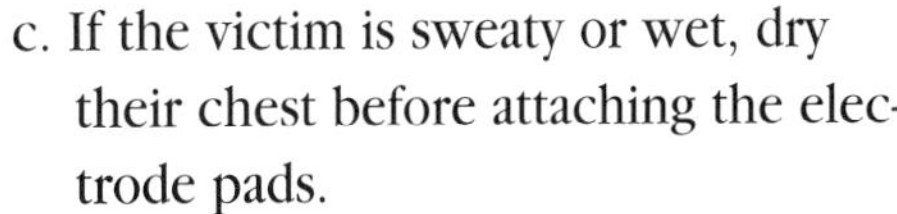

c. If the victim is sweaty or wet, dry their chest before attaching the electrode pads.

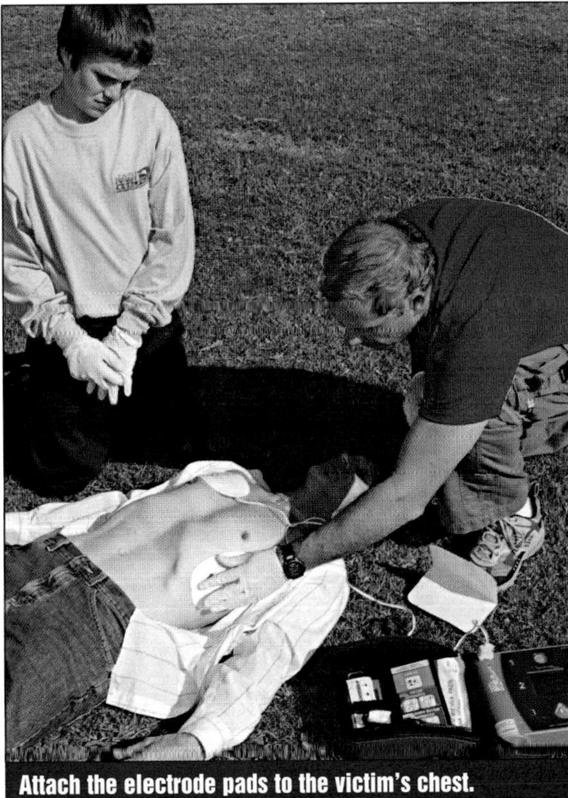
Attach the electrode pads to the victim's chest.

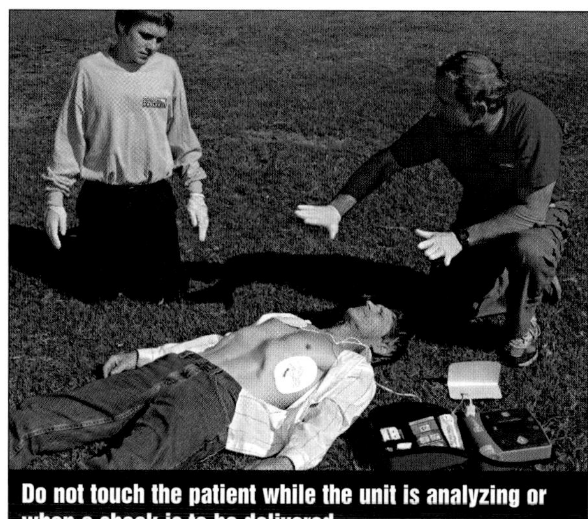

Do not touch the patient while the unit is analyzing or when a shock is to be delivered.

d. If the victim has a hairy chest, press down on the electrode pads firmly for good contact. If this results in a "check electrodes" message, remove the pads (which will remove some of the hair under the pads) and apply a second set of electrode pads. Alternatively, you might have to shave the areas where the electrodes are to be placed.

13. Clear other rescuers and bystanders away from the victim.
14. Press the Analyze button (if necessary) to analyze the victim's heart rhythm for 5 to 15 seconds, depending on the unit.
15. Loudly state "Clear the patient" if a shock is necessary.

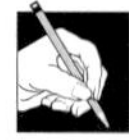

16. Visually check to be sure no one is touching the victim.
17. Press the shock button.
18. Resume CPR for one minute if signs of recovery do not occur.
19. Repeat steps 13 to 18 until signs of recovery are present or medical help arrives to take over.
20. Place the victim in the recovery position, with the AED still attached, if signs of recovery are present.

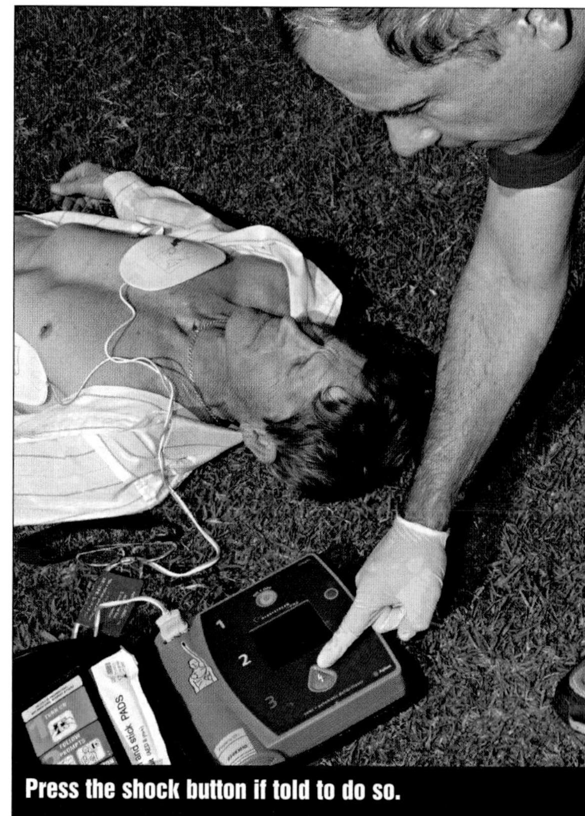

Press the shock button if told to do so.

21. Monitor the victim until medical help arrives.
22. Follow the instructions in the owner's manual of the unit to perform the maintenance needed to ready the unit for its next use.

Note: If administering supplemental oxygen, it is prudent to shut off and move cylinder away from the the patient when using an AED.

REVIEW QUESTIONS

1. The AED should be used within ____________________________ of sudden cardiac arrest (SCA).

2. AED's are always used in conjunction with ____ .

3. In the event that you are ______________ and you have ____________________, leave the victim and retrieve the AED from its storage unit.

4. In the event that you are _____________ and ______________________________ or you know it is ____ give one minute of CPR before leaving the victim to retrieve the AED.

5. The correct placement of the pads is ____ .

6. Before triggering a shock, ____ .

CHAPTER 9

Bleeding

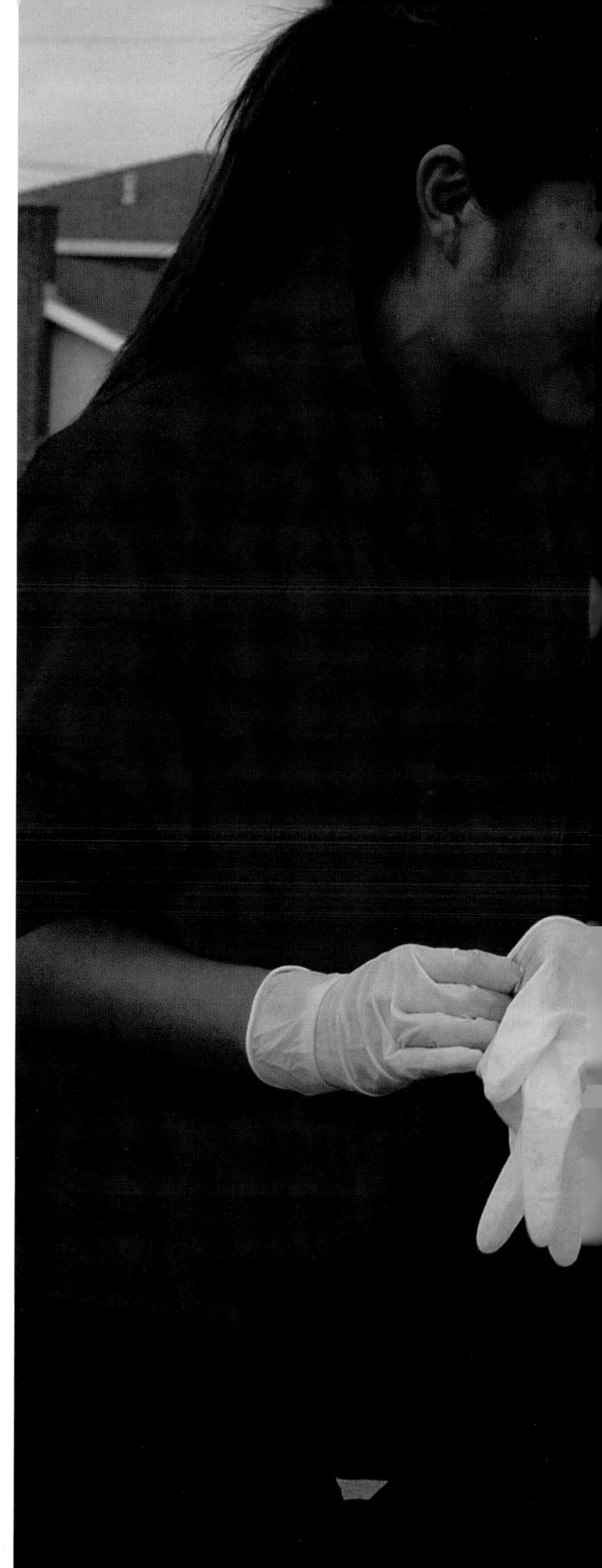

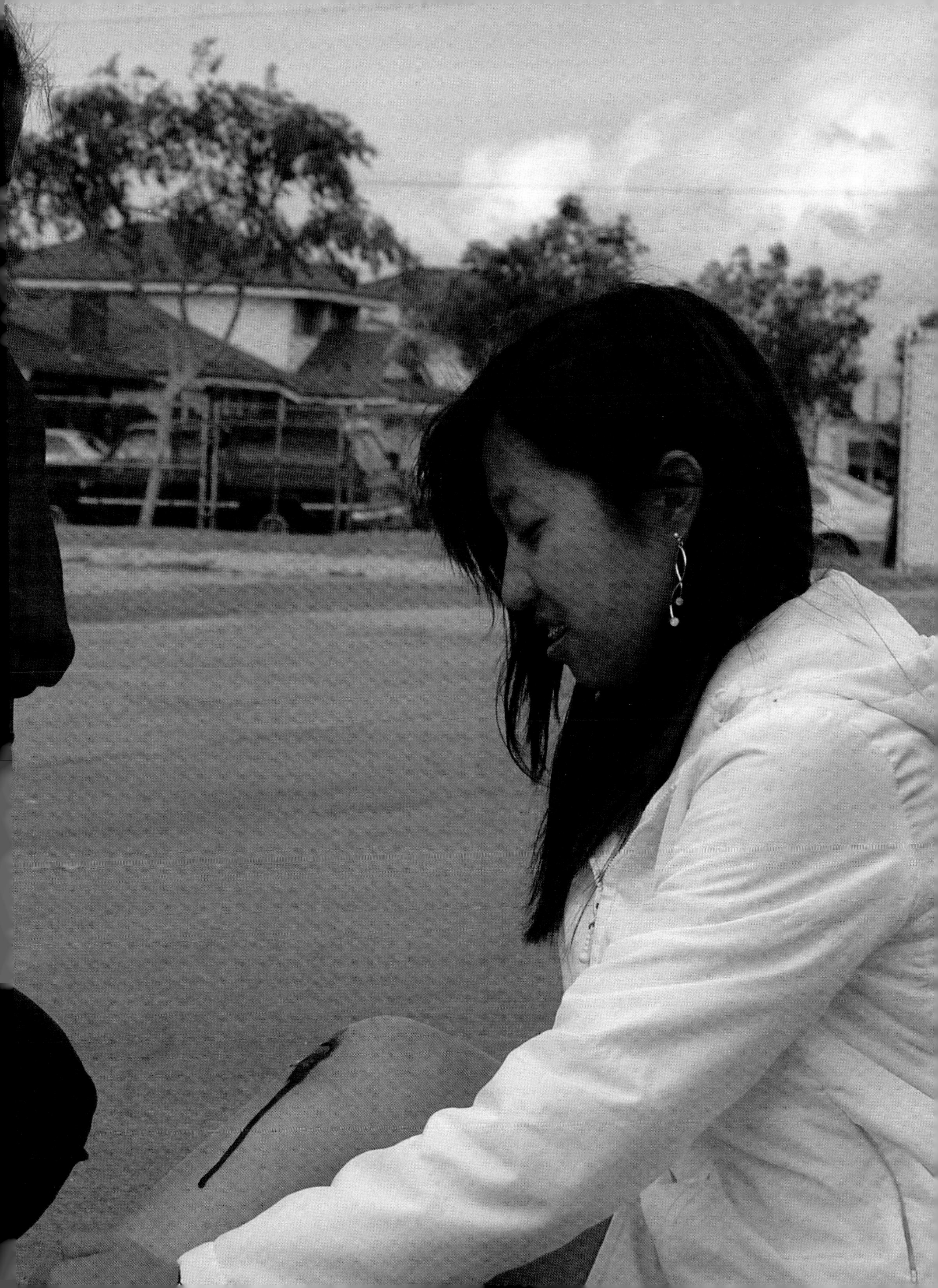

The adult body contains approximately five to six quarts or liters of blood. The body can normally lose one pint (one half liter) of blood without harmful effects. A loss of one quart/liter can cause shock. A loss of two and one half quarts/liters (about half of total blood supply depending on a person's height and weight) usually results in death.

LEARNING GOALS

In this chapter you will learn about:

- Universal precautions as they apply to providing first aid for bleeding
- Types of bleeding: internal vs. external, capillary, arterial, and venous
- Bleeding control: direct pressure, elevation, and pressure points
- Bandaging principles and practice
- Caring for other severe bleeding emergencies: penetrating objects, amputations, internal bleeding

First aid for lesser soft tissue injuries and bleeding will be presented in Chapter 11.

UNIVERSAL PRECAUTIONS

When you encounter a bleeding emergency, you must remember to protect yourself from potentially infected blood. You need to:

- Place a barrier between you and someone else's blood. Latex gloves, protective eye wear, plastic bags, or plastic wrap are all examples of barrier devices.

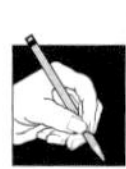

- Cover any open sores, cuts, or scrapes you might have on your hands or exposed skin.
- Minimize the splashing of blood.
- Handle any sharp objects with great care.
- Do not handle any food or drinks when providing first aid.
- Clean and disinfect any area where blood has been spilled using a mixture of one part household bleach to ten parts water.
- Wash your hands and any exposed areas thoroughly, immediately after you have provided first aid or cleaned up a spill.

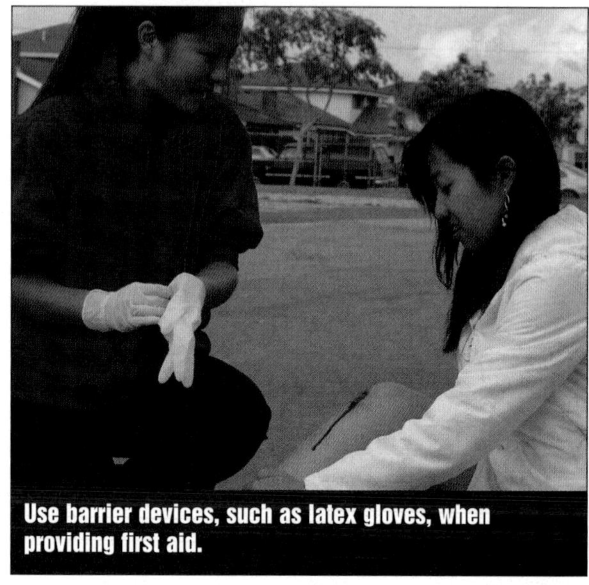

Use barrier devices, such as latex gloves, when providing first aid.

TYPES OF BLEEDING

A bleeding emergency can be from external (open wound) or internal bleeding.

Capillary Bleeding

Capillaries are very small blood vessels that carry blood to and from all parts of the body. Capillary bleeding is slow. The blood oozes from the wound. The body usually can control the bleeding through activating the clotting sequence. Scrapes are one way capillaries get damaged.

Venous Bleeding

Veins are blood vessels that carry blood to the heart. Venous bleeding is dark red or maroon and the blood flows in a steady stream. Cuts or puncture wounds can open veins. You must control venous bleeding. If you do not control venous bleeding, the victim could be placed in a life-threatening situation.

Arterial Bleeding

Arteries are blood vessels that carry blood away from the heart. Arterial bleeding is bright red. The blood spurts from the wound. Arterial bleeding can be life threatening and difficult to control. You must try to control arterial bleeding and get help quickly!

BLEEDING CONTROL

If you need to treat a bleeding injury, use the following steps:

1. Apply direct pressure to the wound. Use a barrier between yourself and the wound.
2. Elevate the injured area.
3. If pressure directly on the wound does not stop the bleeding, apply pressure to the pressure point above the wound. If the wound is on the arm, apply pressure to the brachial artery by compressing the artery against the humerus (upper arm bone) with your fingers. If the wound is on the leg, apply pressure to the femoral artery by compressing the artery against the pelvic bone with the heel of your hand.

Bandaging and Dressing

Dressings are sterile pads put directly on the wound to soak up the blood, quell further bleeding when pressure is applied, and protect the wound from further contamination. Gauze pads are one common type of dressing. You use bandages to hold the dressings in place and to apply pressure to the wound to help stop the bleeding. Bandages are any material you use to wrap or cover and immobilize the wound. Some common types of bandages are adhesive bandages, roller bandages, and elastic bandages.

Skill Performance

You use a pressure dressing and bandage to help control bleeding. The steps to apply a pressure dressing and bandage are:

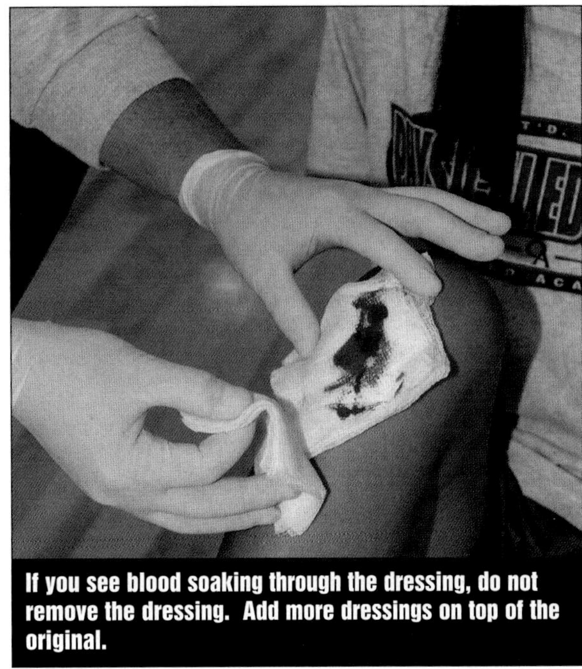

If you see blood soaking through the dressing, do not remove the dressing. Add more dressings on top of the original.

1. Place a sterile dressing on the wound.
2. Apply pressure to the dressing and elevate the extremity higher than the victim's heart.
3. If you see blood soaking through the dressing, do not remove the dressing. Add more dressings on top of the original.
4. When bleeding has been controlled, apply a bandage to hold the dressing in place and maintain pressure on the wound.
5. Hold the end of the roller bandage on one side of the dressing.
6. Wrap the bandage around the wound, using overlapping turns to cover the dressing completely.
7. Tie or tape the bandage in place.
8. Check the fingers or toes beyond the bandage for evidence of circulation. Press gently on the nail. The nail bed should lighten,and upon, color should rapidly return. The fingers or toes should have good color. They should not be gray or blue in color.

If you still see blood soaking through the bandage, do not remove the bandage. Add more dressings on top of the original bandage and secure with another roller bandage.

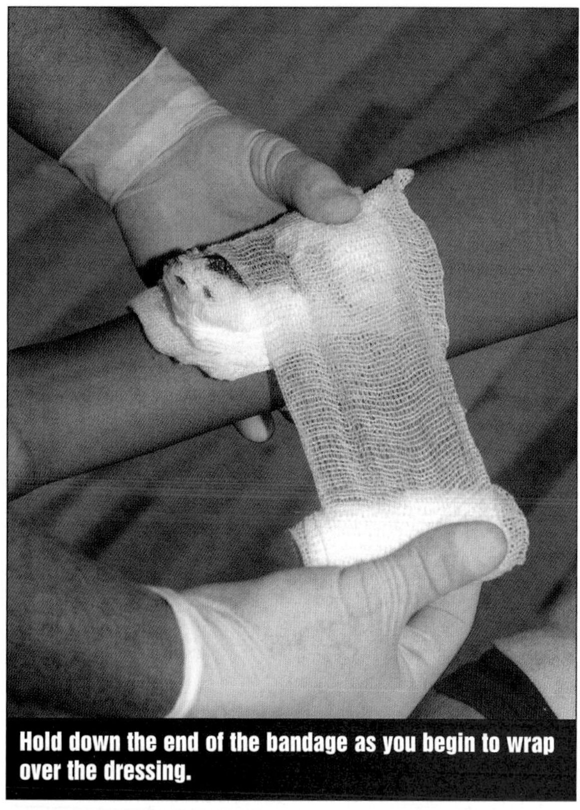

Hold down the end of the bandage as you begin to wrap over the dressing.

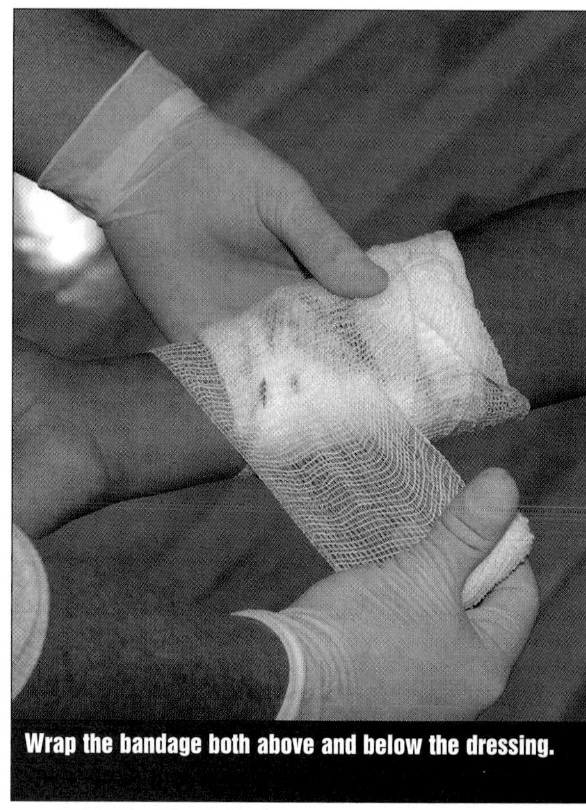

Wrap the bandage both above and below the dressing.

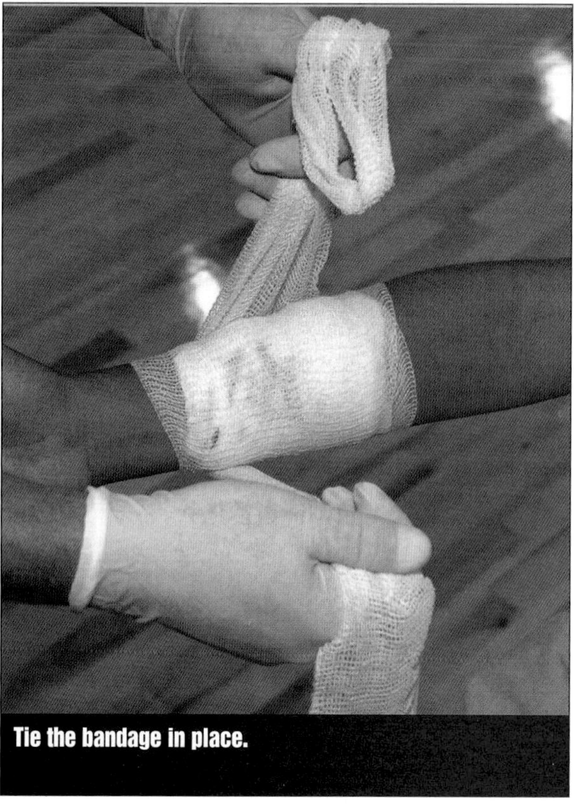

Tie the bandage in place.

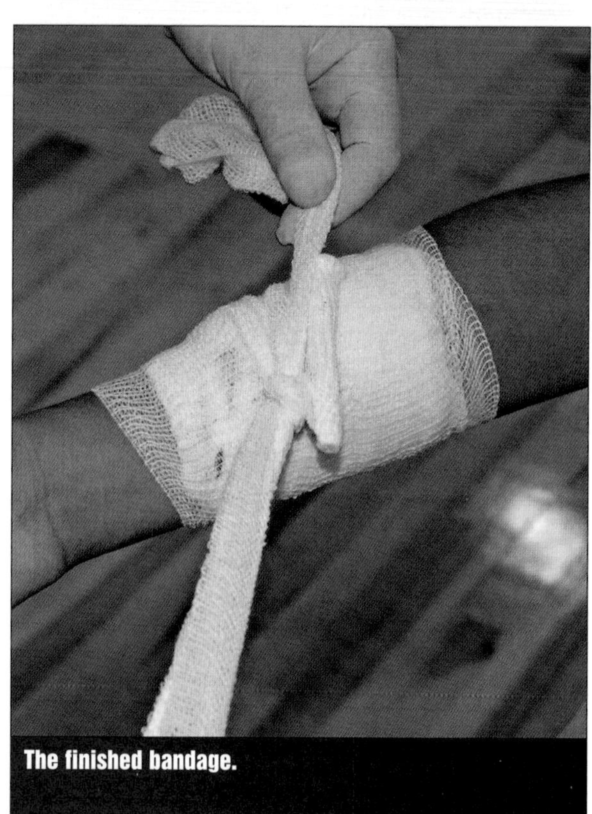

The finished bandage.

OTHER BLEEDING EMERGENCIES

You may also see bleeding emergencies where the victim has an object piercing their body, a part of their body is missing, or they have internal bleeding.

Penetrating Objects

If the victim has the object (such as a knife or piece of glass) that caused the wound still in their body, do not try to remove it as it will likely cause more tissue damage or bleeding. Bandage around the object to stabilize it. Also, keep the victim from unnecessarily moving.

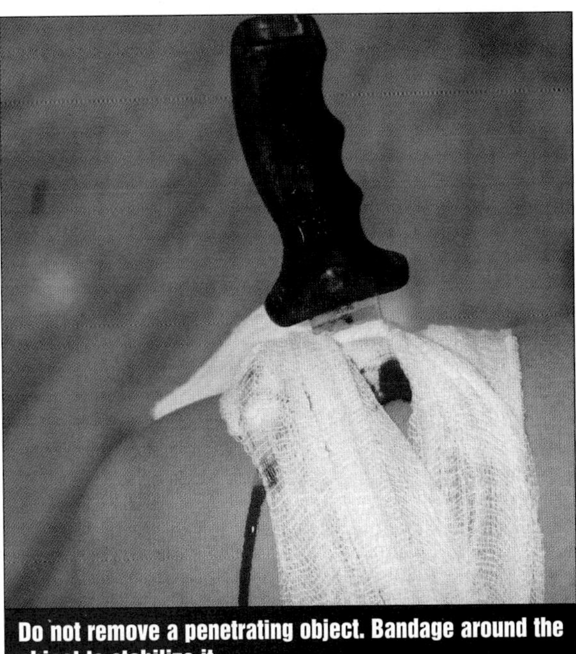

Do not remove a penetrating object. Bandage around the object to stabilize it.

Amputations

If you need to treat a victim with an amputated body part, use the following steps:

1. Follow the steps for bleeding control.
2. Find the missing body part (if possible) and wrap it in a sterile or clean cloth.
3. Place the body part in a plastic bag and seal it.
4. Place the bag on a bed of ice. Do not cover the bag in ice.
5. Be sure the body part is transported to the hospital with the victim.

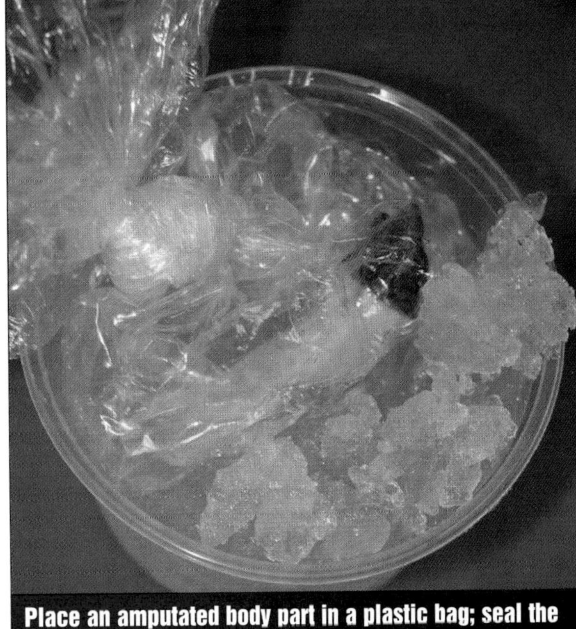

Place an amputated body part in a plastic bag; seal the bag and place it on a bed of ice.

INTERNAL BLEEDING

You might have a victim who is bleeding internally. The signs and symptoms of internal bleeding can include:

- Blood loss from the mouth, nose, ear, rectum, vagina, or urinary tract
- A painful, tender, or hard area on the chest or abdomen
- Rapid and weak pulse
- Cool or moist skin
- Purplish bruising and swelling of the damaged area
- Person has feeling of dread or something being wrong

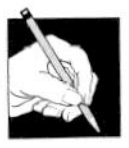

If you suspect internal bleeding, do the following:

1. Treat for shock.
2. Be alert for vomiting.
3. Apply an ice pack to the damaged area, with a cloth between the ice and the victim's skin.

REVIEW QUESTIONS

1. ____

are all examples of barrier devices.

2. Capillary bleeding is ____ .

3. Venous bleeding is ____________________ and the blood ____________________.

4. Arterial bleeding is ________________ and the blood ____________ from the wound.

5. If you need to treat a bleeding emergency, use the following steps - summarize the steps from the text - ____

____ .

6. You use bandages to ____________________ and to ____________________ to the wound to help stop the bleeding.

7. If the victim has the object (such as a knife or piece of glass) that caused the wound still in their body, ____ .

8. If you need to treat a victim with an amputated body part - list the steps from the text.

____

____

____

____

____

9. If you suspect internal bleeding, do the following - list the steps from the text.

____

____

____

Notes

CHAPTER 10

Shock

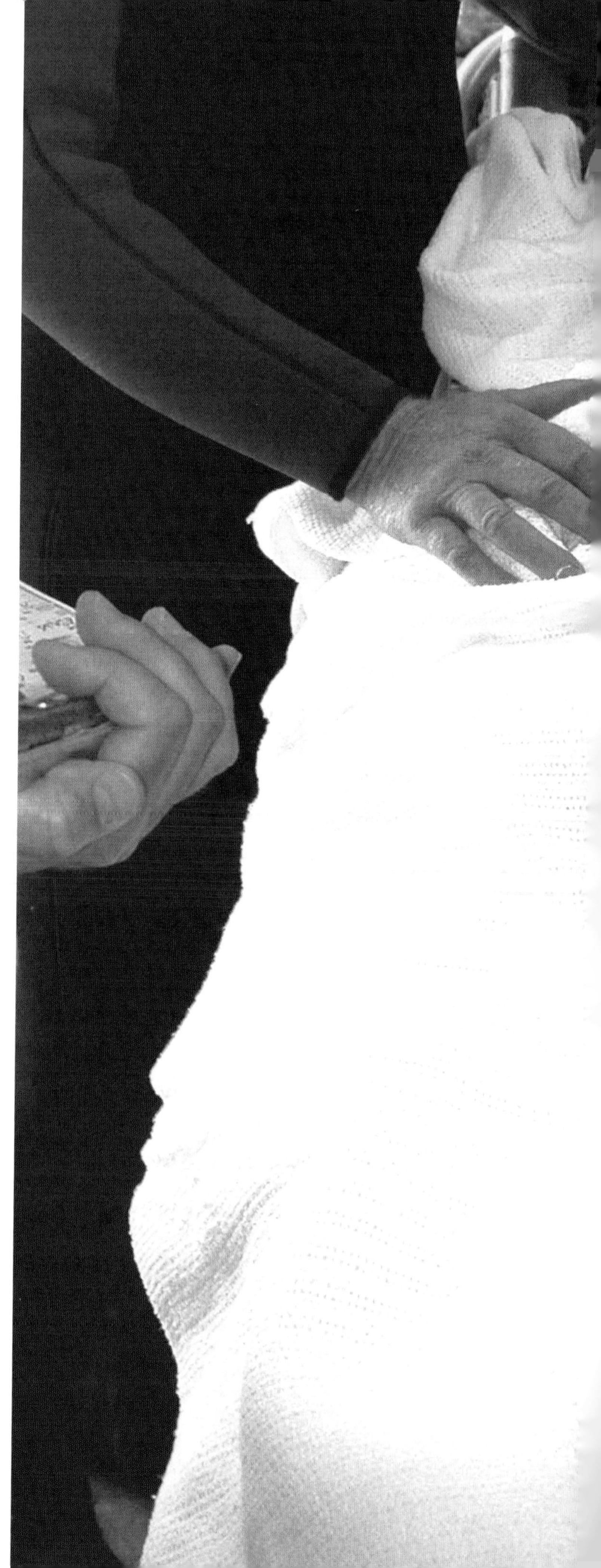

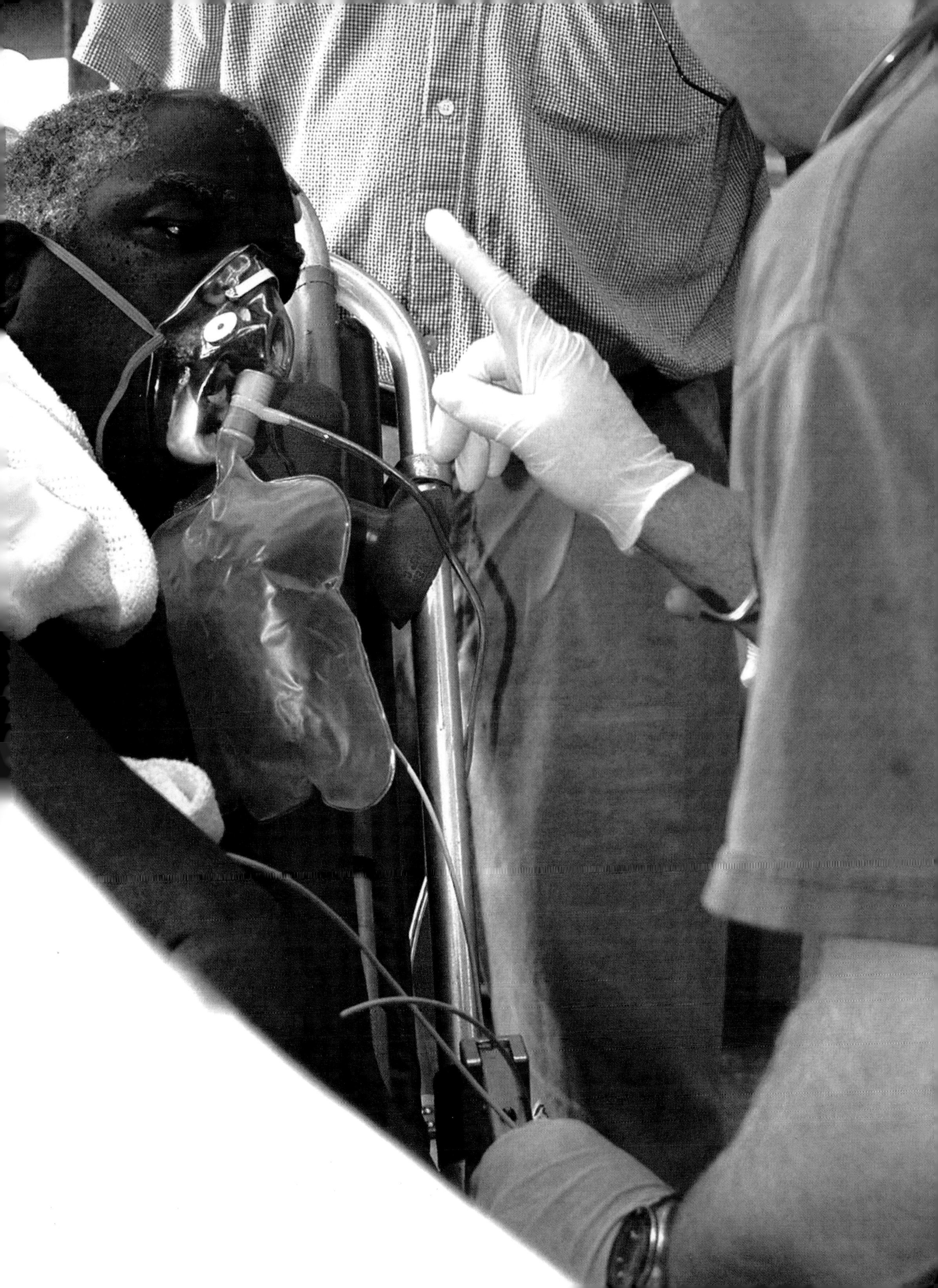

Shock can occur even in the absence of any apparent injury. For example, fainting is a form of shock. Shock is a condition that occurs whenever the circulatory system fails to deliver an adequate blood supply to all areas of the body. Whenever you treat a victim for any injury, you also want to treat them for shock.

LEARNING GOALS

In this chapter you will learn about:

- Causes of shock
- Signs/symptoms of shock
- Care for shock

CAUSES OF SHOCK

Shock is the failure of the heart and blood vessels to maintain enough oxygen-rich blood flowing to the vital organs of the body. There is some degree of shock with almost every illness or injury.

Shock can bc life threatening. You need to recognize the signs and symptoms and to begin treating the victim before shock completely develops. It is unlikely that you will see all the signs and symptoms of shock in a single victim. Sometimes the signs and symptoms are disguised by the illness or injury or they might not appear immediately. In fact, many times the symptoms appear hours later.

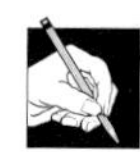

Hypovolemic shock is caused by a decreased amount of blood or fluids in the body. This decrease results from injuries that produce internal and external bleeding, fluid loss due to burns, and dehydration due to severe vomiting and diarrhea. **Neurogenic shock** is caused by an abnormal enlargement of the blood vessels and pooling of the blood to a degree that adequate blood flow cannot be maintained. **Septic shock** occurs when toxins produced by certain bacteria have an effect on the body that lowers effective perfusion. **Psychogenic shock** is a shock-like condition produced by excessive fear, joy, anger, or grief. Where these conditions reduce blood pressure, the reduced circulating volume can become deficient and result in shock.

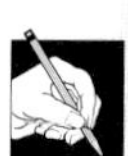

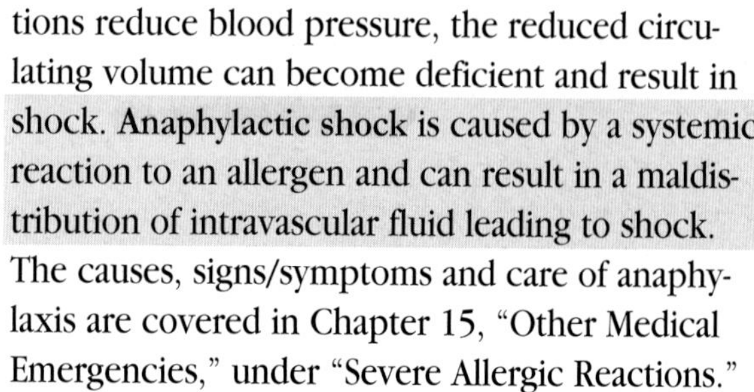

Anaphylactic shock is caused by a systemic reaction to an allergen and can result in a maldistribution of intravascular fluid leading to shock. The causes, signs/symptoms and care of anaphylaxis are covered in Chapter 15, "Other Medical Emergencies," under "Severe Allergic Reactions."

SIGNS AND SYMPTOMS OF SHOCK

The signs and symptoms of shock include:

- Weakness
- Fainting, faintness
- Pale, cool, and moist skin
- Rapid pulse rate
- Thirst
- Anxiety, restlessness, or irritability
- Nausea
- Altered consciousness
- Dazed expression and a blank look on the facc

CARE FOR SHOCK

Caring for shock includes the following techniques:

- Have the victim lie down.
- Elevate their legs 10 to 12 inches (25 to 30 centimeters), unless you suspect a spinal injury, chest or abdominal injury, or broken leg or pelvic bones.
- Make the victim as comfortable as possible. With the victim's permission, loosen any restricting clothing. Talk to them in a calm and reassuring tone to help relieve stress and anxiety. A good "bed-side manner" is frequently the most effective care. Handle the victim gently.
- Maintain the victim's body temperature. Cover them with a blanket and insulate them from ground, if necessary to prevent heat loss or against heat gain when heat is a factor.

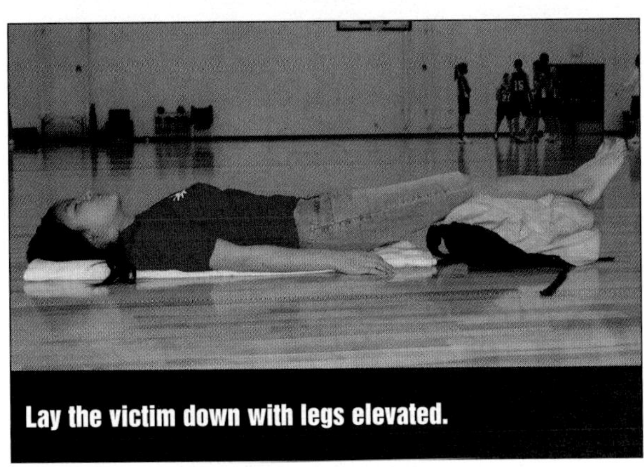
Lay the victim down with legs elevated.

- Provide the victim with plenty of fresh air by controlling bystanders and clearing the immediate area to allow air flow. If you are trained to do so, administer supplemental oxygen, if available.
- Do not give victims anything to eat or drink because they may be nauseated and vomit or they may be allergic to what you give them.
- If victims become nauseated, turn them onto their side in case they start vomiting-unless their injury prevents it.

REVIEW QUESTIONS

1. ______________________________ is caused by a decreased amount of blood or fluids in the body.
2. ______________________________ is caused by an abnormal enlargement of the blood vessels and pooling of the blood to a degree that adequate blood flow cannot be maintained.
3. ______________________________ occurs when toxins produced by certain bacteria have an effect on the body that lowers effective perfusion.
4. ______________________________ is a shock-like condition produced by excessive fear, joy, anger, or grief.
5. ______________________________ is caused by a systemic reaction to an allergen and can result in a maldistribution of intravascular fluid leading to shock.
6. The signs and symptoms of shock include: - list 5 of the 9 signs and symptoms from the text.

____

____

____

____

7. Caring for shock includes the several techniques: - list 4 of the 7 techniques from the text.

____

____

____

____

CHAPTER 11

Soft Tissue Injuries

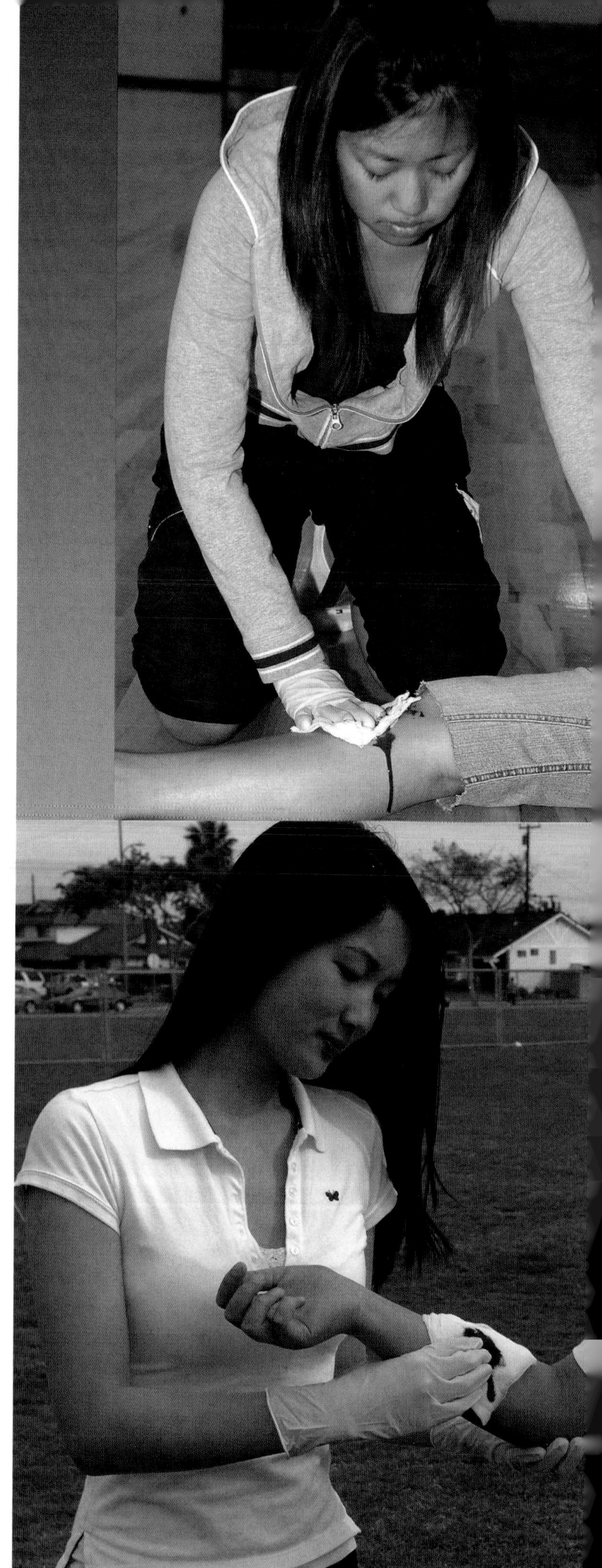

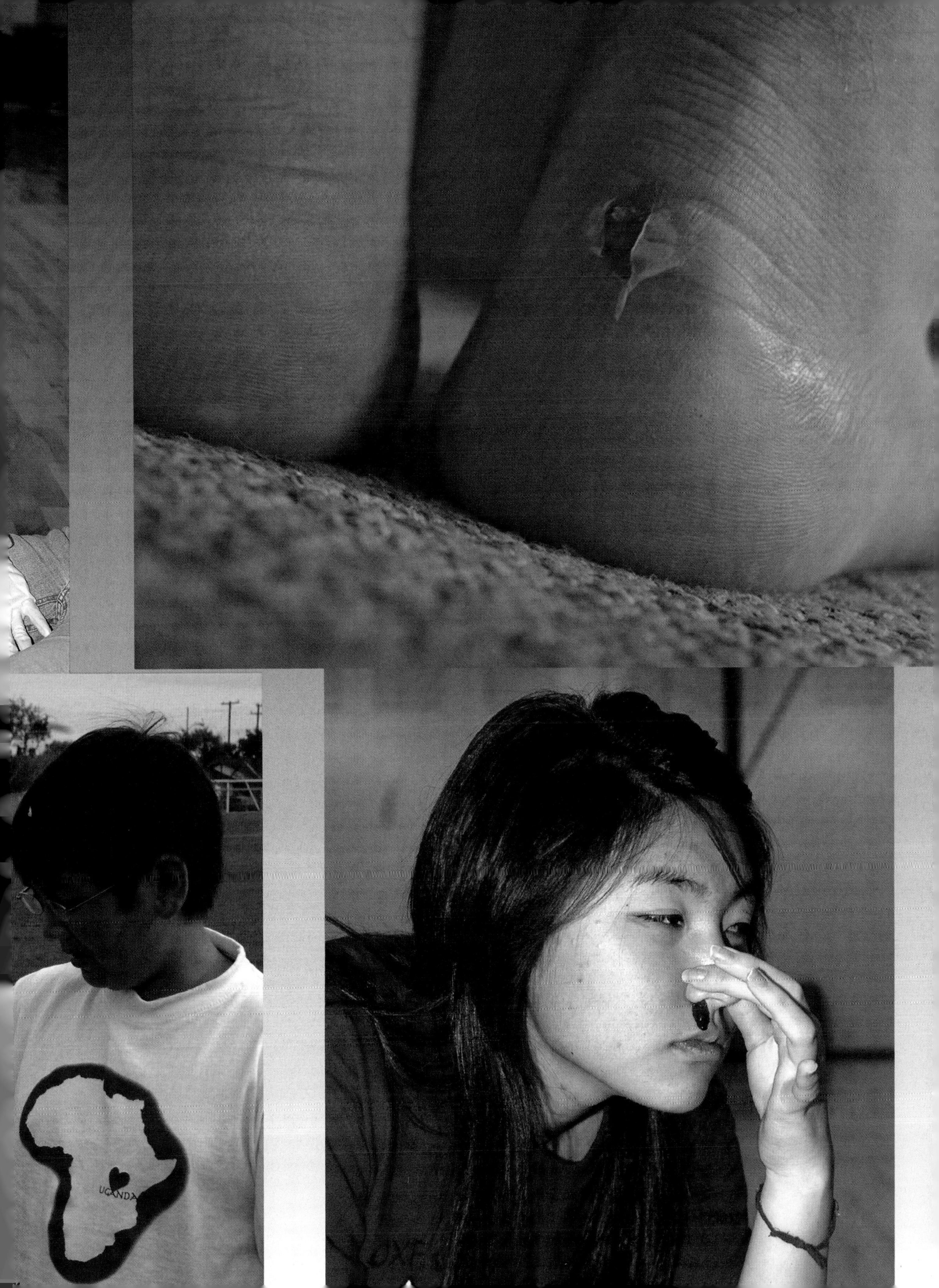
UGANDA

The soft tissue injuries discussed in this chapter are typically not serious and proper first aid can prevent complications from infection and hasten the healing process. First aid for serious bleeding injuries was presented in Chapter 9.

LEARNING GOALS

In this chapter you will learn about:

- Closed soft tissue injuries including bruises, contusions, hematomas, blisters, eye injuries, nose bleeds and abdominal injuries
- Open soft tissue injuries including blisters, abrasions, lacerations, incisions and punctures

CLOSED SOFT TISSUE INJURIES

Bruises (Contusions and Hematomas)

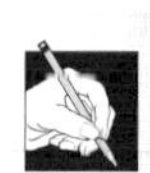

Bruises (also called contusions) occur when you have a blow to a muscle or other soft tissue. The blow damages the blood vessels, causing bleeding and swelling. At first, the area appears red and then darkens to purple and other colors like yellow over time. A large or painful bruise can be a sign of severe damage to deep tissues.

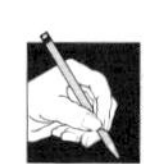

A hematoma is a term for a localized collection of blood (usually clotted) and usually situated within an organ or a soft tissue space. It is also a term used by lay persons interchangeably with bruise and contusion. There are many types of hematomas and they are named depending on their location on or in the body, for example a subdural hematoma is located on the surface of the brain inside the skull and can be life threatening, whereas an subungual hematoma is under a finger or toe nail and may result in the loss of the nail, but if infected, could become serious. A hematoma auris is also known as a cauliflower ear. Hematomas may be obvious, as in the latter examples, or not so, when they occur internally. First aid for suspected concussion and head injuries is described later in this chapter. For minor hematomas, contusions, and bruises the recommended first aid is as follows.

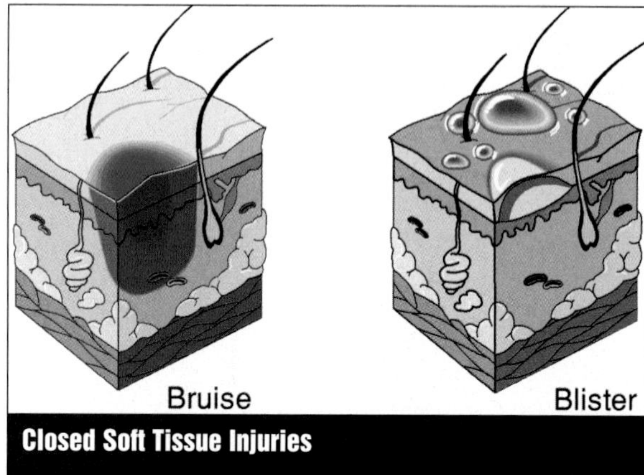

Closed Soft Tissue Injuries

First Aid for Bruises (Contusions and Hematomas)

Use the following steps to care for a bruise:

1. Get the victim into a comfortable, resting position.
2. Elevate the injured area.
3. Apply an ice pack to the injured area. Place a cloth for insulation between any plastic ice pack and the skin.
4. Wrap the injured area with a bandage to hold the ice pack in place. Do not wrap the bandage too tightly.
5. Monitor for shock.
6. Transport to medical care, if necessary.

Blisters

Blisters usually form because of friction, sunburn, and second degree burns from a heat source. It is the body's natural defense that allows the damaged skin to heal itself in a sterile environment. Do not break a blister. Use the following steps if someone has an unbroken blister:

1. Gently wash the area around the blister.
2. Cut a hole in several gauze pads and tape the gauze over the blistered area with the hole over the blister.

Use the following steps if someone has a broken blister:

1. Gently wash the area around the blister.
2. Cover the area with a sterile gauze and tape the gauze in place.

Eye Injuries

Any injury to the eye requires medical attention. Use the following steps if someone has sustained a blow or penetrating injury to their eye:

1. Use an eye shield or place padding around the eye to prevent pressure on the injured eyeball. The padding can be fashioned from a stack of several gauze pads with a hole cut in the middle or a donut-shaped twist of cloth. Bandage the protective shield in place.
2. If the penetrating object is still present, do not remove it. Use a paper cup or cone over the object and secure it in place. This will keep the object from being disturbed.
3. Place a patch over the other eye and bandage it in place to prevent eye movement. (The eyes move together, and the injured eye will follow any movement of the uninjured eye.)
4. Seek medical attention.

Use the following steps if chemicals have gotten into someone's eye:

1. Flood the eye with warm water. Flood the eye in a downward direction and away from the nose.
2. Encourage the person to look around in order to roll their own eye as much as possible while flooding the eye with water.
3. Seek medical attention.

Use the following steps if a small non-penetrating object is in someone's eye (dirt, eyelash, etc.):

1. Irrigate the eye with an eyewash or warm water while turning the affected eye down, so you don't wash particles into the other eye.
2. If this is unsuccessful, hold a cotton swab or small stick horizontally against the top of the upper eyelid, grasp the eyelid, and fold it up over the swab.
3. Inspect the undersurface of the lid for the object, and gently wipe it away with moistened gauze. Do not touch the cornea.
4. If you do not see the object, pull the lower eyelid down, inspect between the lower eyelid and the eye, and gently wipe the object away if it is seen.
5. If the victim still feels some irritation, patch the eye closed.
6. If the irritation remains after 24 hours, seek medical attention.

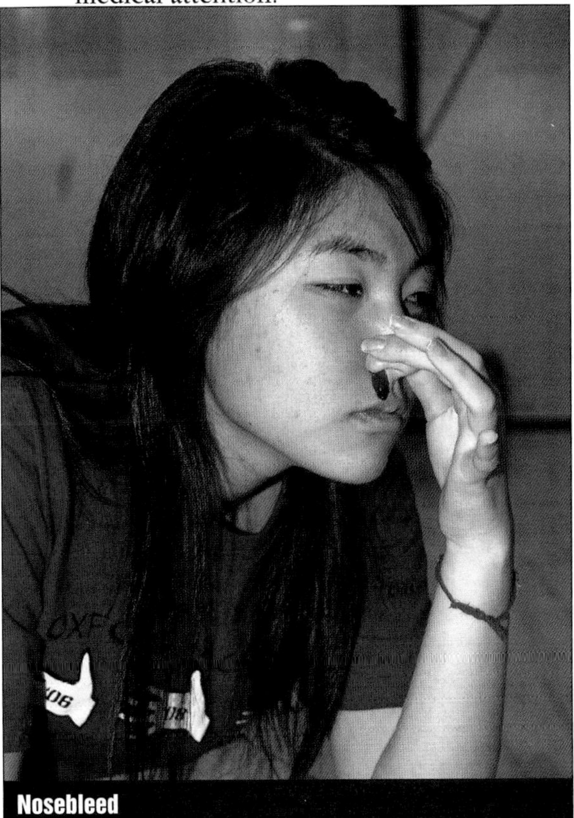

Nosebleed

Nosebleed

Nosebleeds are usually caused by a blow to the nose. High blood pressure, medication especially Coumadin® (a blood thinner), and changes in altitude can also cause nosebleeds. Use the following steps if someone has a nosebleed:

1. Have the victim sit down with their head tilted slightly forward.
2. Have the victim control the bleeding through one of the following methods:
    - Pinching their nostrils together and holding it for 10 minutes by the clock.
    - Applying an ice pack to the bridge of the nose. Place a cloth for insulation between any plastic ice pack and the skin.
    - Putting pressure on the upper lip just beneath the nose.
3. If the bleeding does not stop or you suspect that the victim has a broken nose, seek medical attention.

Abdominal Injuries

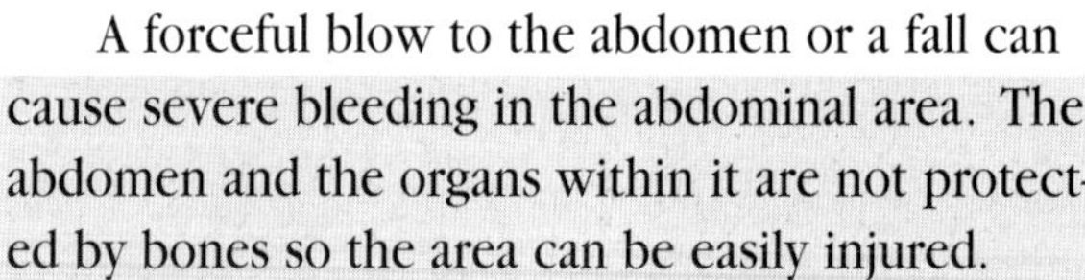

A forceful blow to the abdomen or a fall can cause severe bleeding in the abdominal area. The abdomen and the organs within it are not protected by bones so the area can be easily injured. Use the following steps if someone has received a blow to the abdomen:

1. Help the victim lie flat. You can bend their knees slightly to make the victim more comfortable.
2. Call for help.
3. Look for signs of internal bleeding:
    - Tenderness, swelling, or bruising in the abdominal area
    - Rapid, weak pulse
    - Cool or moist skin that looks pale or blue
    - Vomiting or coughing up blood
    - Excessive thirst
    - Confusion, drowsiness, fainting, or unconsciousness
4. Treat for shock.
5. Do not give the victim anything to drink or eat.

Use the following steps if the injury to the abdomen has opened a wound and organs are exposed:

1. Help the victim lie flat.
2. Call for help.
3. Do not apply pressure to the organs or attempt to push them back into the abdominal cavity.
4. Remove any clothing around the wound.
5. If the wound is from a penetrating object, and it is still present, put padding around the object to stabilize it and prevent any movement.
6. Place moist sterile dressings or wet, clean cloths over the wound or exposed organs. Use warm tap water to moisten the dressings.
7. Treat for shock.

There are many causes of severe abdominal pain that are not related to injury. These can include:

- Ulcers
- Stomach flu
- Hepatitis
- Gallstones
- Appendicitis
- Disorders of pregnancy
- Kidney stone
- Bowel obstruction
- Hernia
- Diarrhea

The pain can be sharp, cramp-like, or aching. It can be localized or widespread. There can be nausea, vomiting, or diarrhea. The interview of the victim might reveal that they have had a similar episode previously and were given a specific diagnosis. Use the following steps if someone is suffering severe abdominal pain:

1. Help the victim lie down in a comfortable position. You can bend their knees slightly to make the victim more comfortable.
2. Call for help.
3. Treat for shock.

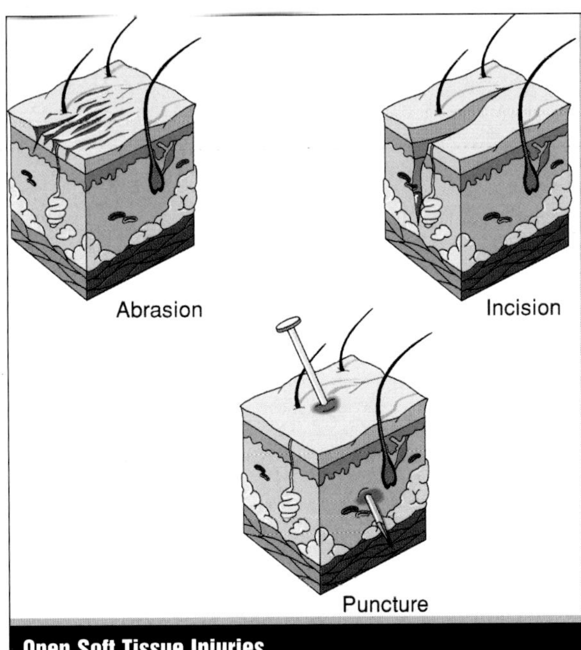

Open Soft Tissue Injuries

OPEN SOFT TISSUE INJURIES

Abrasions

An abrasion is a wearing down of the outer layers of the skin by friction, as in a "skinned knee." Bleeding is usually not severe, but the wound can be very painful and can easily become infected. Use the following steps if someone has an abrasion.

1. Gently wash the wounded area thoroughly with soap and water.
2. Wash away any dirt or other foreign matter from the wound site.
3. Cover with sterile non-adhesive dressing and bandage.

Lacerations and Incisions

A laceration is a torn ragged wound whereas an incision is a "clean" cut, usually caused by a sharp bladed instrument like a knife or razor blade. Lacerations and incisions can be minor with very little bleeding or severe and life-threatening. In the event of severe lacerations or incisions, controlling bleeding and advanced care are a priority. Use the following steps if someone has a minor laceration or incision.

1. Gently wash the wounded area thoroughly with soap and water.
2. Wash away any dirt or other foreign matter from the wound site.
3. Cover with a sterile dressing and apply direct pressure to stop the bleeding.
4. Bandage the sterile dressing in place.

Punctures

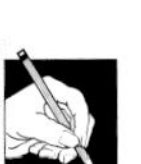

Puncture wounds are caused by sharp objects like nails and easily become infected. Thorough cleansing of the wound is important. Severe puncture wounds (impalement) require medical attention. Follow the steps listed above in Chapter 9 or under "Chest Wounds" (Chapter 12) until medical assistance is obtained.

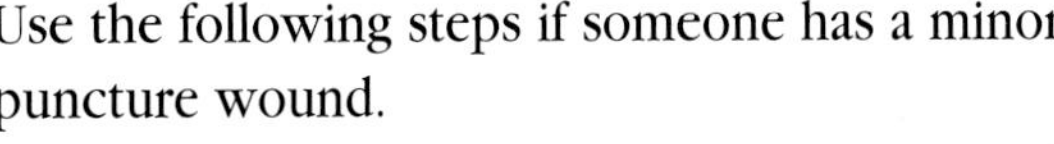

Use the following steps if someone has a minor puncture wound.

1. Gently wash the wounded area thoroughly with soap and water.
2. Wash away any dirt or other foreign matter from the wound site. If possible position the wound so that a stream of clean water will flow into the top edge of the puncture and out of the bottom side of the wound to aid in the removal of foreign matter and infectious bacteria.
3. Cover with a sterile dressing and apply direct pressure to stop the bleeding.
4. Bandage a sterile dressing in place.

Bandaging and Dressing

See Chapter 9 for information on bandaging and dressing.

REVIEW QUESTIONS

1. Bruises (also called contusions) occur when you have a ______________________________ __________. The _______ damages the blood vessels, causing ______________________ ____.

2. A hematoma is a term for a _________________________________ and usually situated ____

3. ______________________ a blister.

4. Use the following steps if someone has sustained a blow or penetrating injury to their eye: List 2 of the steps from the text. ____ ____.

5. The abdomen and the organs within it are ________________________ so the area can be ____.

6. An abrasion is a ____ by friction.

7. A _________ is a torn ragged wound whereas an ______________ is a "clean" cut, usually caused by a sharp bladed instrument like a knife or razor blade.

8. Puncture wounds are caused by sharp objects like nails and _________________________ ____ of the wound is important.

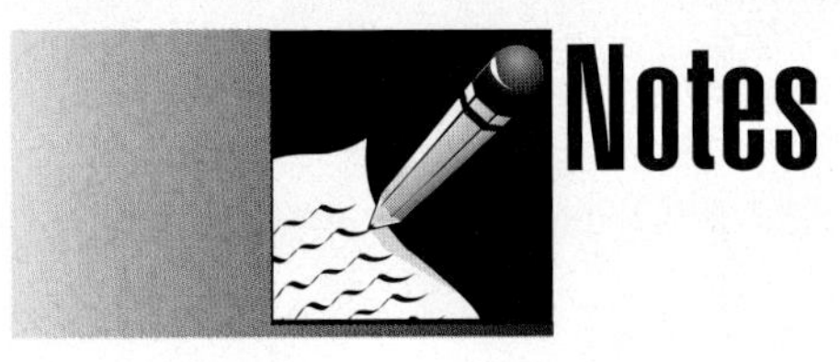

Notes

CHAPTER 12

Musculoskeletal Injuries

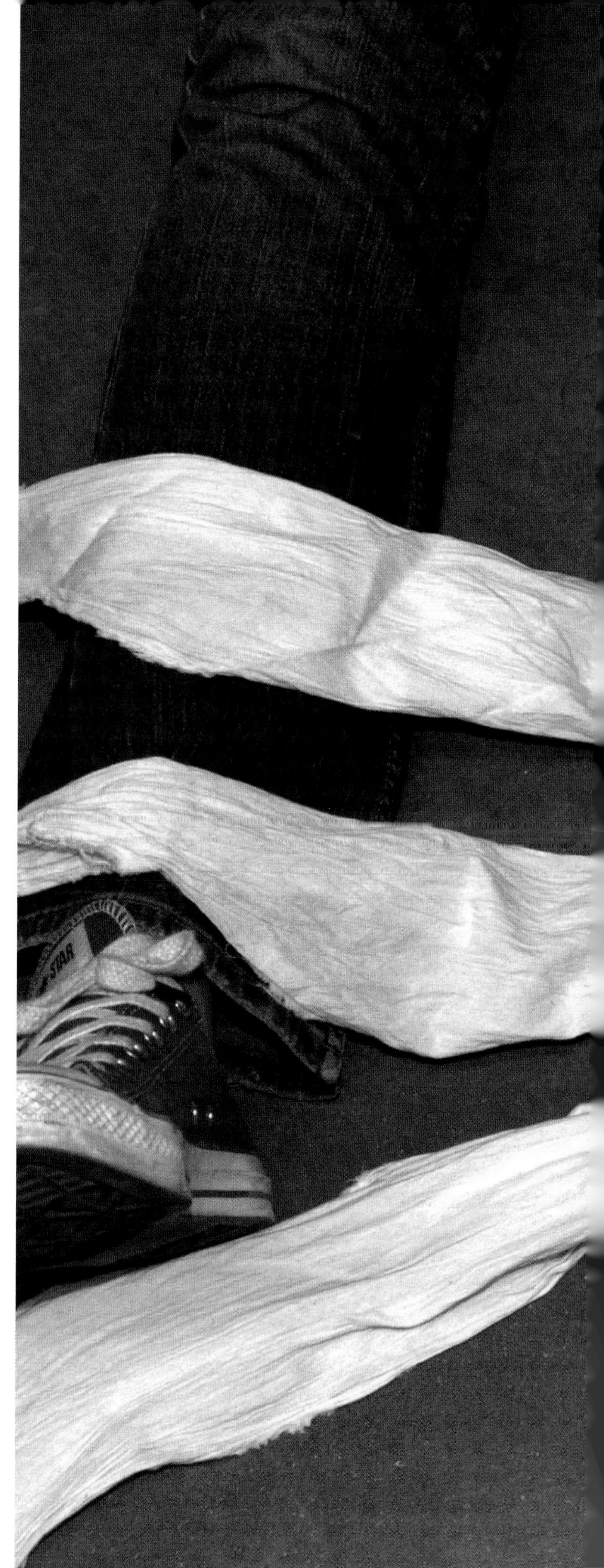

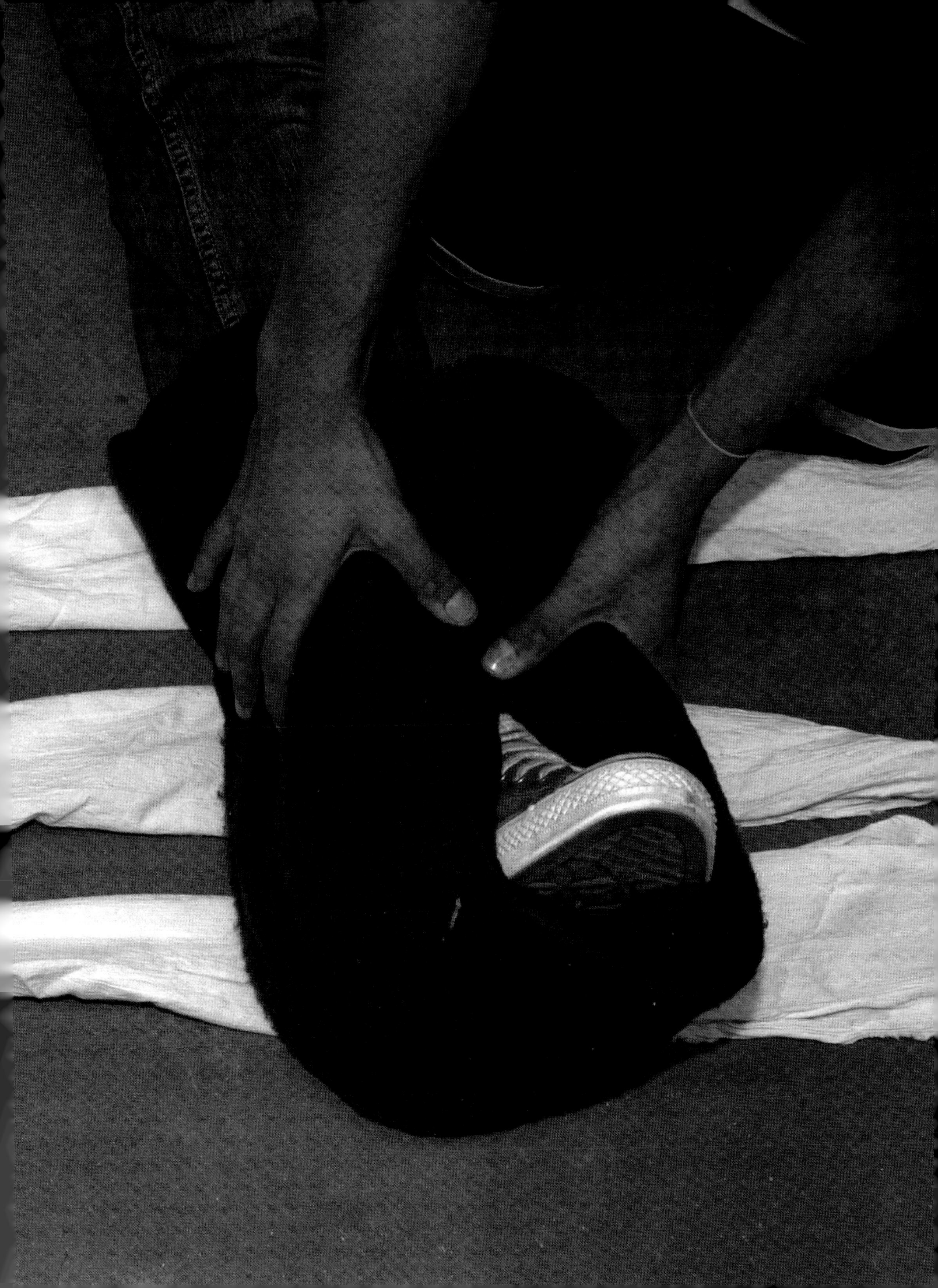

The musculoskeletal system includes all the bones, muscles, tendons, ligaments, joints, cartilage, and other connective tissue in the body. Injuries to muscles and joints are common occurrences. They can happen at work, at home, or during leisure time. Although rarely life-threatening, they are painful and may sometimes lead to a long-term decrease in function, particularly if not handled well from the start. Other injuries to the musculoskeletal system can be severe and result in lifelong disability, as in the case of spinal cord injuries. In the latter instance proper first aid can mitigate the long term consequences associated with these injuries.

LEARNING GOALS

In this chapter you will learn about:

- Head, neck, and spinal injuries
- Chest injuries
- Injures of the extremities - strains and sprains, dislocations, and fractures
- Splinting Principles and Practice Skill Performance
- Special considerations: "crushing" injuries

HEAD AND NECK INJURIES

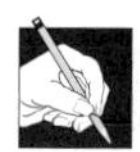

There are two types of head injuries:

- Open
- Closed

With open head injuries, you will see bleeding wounds to the face or head. The scalp is very vascular and there is often a lot of bleeding. With a closed head injury, you will see no visible signs of injury to the face or head. Signs and symptoms of a closed head injury include:

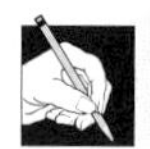

- Loss of consciousness
- Confusion
- Drowsiness
- Clear fluid draining from the ears or nose
- Compressions or deformities to the skull
- Black eyes or bruised skin behind one or both ears
- Double or blurred vision
- Unequal pupils
- Nausea or vomiting

Use the following steps if someone has a head injury and is conscious:

1. Call for help.
2. If the person is leaking clear fluid from ear or nose, pad the affected ear, and gently turn the victim to the affected side.
3. If the person has a bleeding wound, place a dressing on the wound and gently apply direct pressure.

Use the following steps if someone has a head injury and is unconscious:

1. Call for help.
2. Check for airway, breathing, and circulation, and start CPR if necessary.
3. If the person is leaking clear fluid from ear, pad the affected ear, and gently turn the victim to the affected side.
4. If the person has a bleeding wound, place a dressing on the wound and gently apply direct pressure.

CONCUSSION

A concussion is caused by a significant blow to the head and may result in a brief period of unconsciousness (for less than five minutes). Use the following steps if someone has sustained a blow to the head:

1. Help the person lie down, with their shoulders and head slightly elevated.
2. Control any bleeding.
3. Check for signs of a serious head injury.
4. Transport the victim to medical attention.
5. Be alert for any danger signs over the next two days. These danger signs include:
   - Persistent vomiting
   - Loss of coordination
   - Severe headaches

SPINAL INJURIES

Injuries to the neck (cervical vertebrae), or spine (thoracic, lumbar, sacral, and coccyx vertebrae) can be disabling to the victim. You should always suspect a neck, or spinal injury in any of the following situations:

- An automobile accident
- An ejection from an automobile
- An accident diving into a body of water
- Surfing or body surfing
- A fall from a height greater than the victim's personal height
- A victim found unconscious for an unknown reason or in an unnatural or awkward position
- A severe blow to the head, neck, or back
- A lightning strike
- A gunshot wound to the head, neck, or trunk of the body
- Any injury in which the victim's protective head-gear (helmet) is broken

Look for the following signs and symptoms of a head, neck, or spinal injury:

- Changes in consciousness
- Cool or clammy skin
- Severe pain or pressure in the head, neck, or back
- Tingling or numbness in the hands, fingers, feet, or toes
- Partial or total paralysis of any body part
- Difficulty breathing
- Impaired vision
- Vomiting
- Loss of balance
- Any unusual bumps or depressions in the head, neck, or spinal area
- Blood or clear fluid draining from the ear
- Seizures

If you do suspect a neck or spinal injury, use the following steps:

1. Call for help
2. Minimize movement of the victim's head and spine by placing your hands on both sides of the victim's head and holding their head in line with their body until help arrives.
3. Monitor the victim for breathing (using the jaw lift method if necessary) and circulation.
4. Control any external bleeding.
5. Treat for shock.

DENTAL INJURIES

Injuries to the teeth need to be treated by a dentist as soon as possible. These injuries can include toothaches, broken or lost teeth, lost fillings, or infections. Use the following steps to care for someone who has had a tooth knocked out:

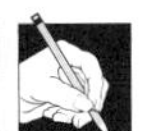

1. Have the victim sit with their head tilted slightly forward to allow blood to drain from the mouth.
2. Roll a sterile dressing and place it in the space left by the missing tooth. Have the victim bite down to keep the dressing in place.
3. Treat the tooth in one of the following ways:
   - Pick up the tooth by the crown, rinse it in cool water, and place it back in the socket.
   - Place the tooth in a small container of milk.
4. Take the victim and the tooth to the dentist or an emergency room as soon as possible. The tooth must be replaced within 30 minutes and receive care from a dentist as soon as possible.

Use the following steps to care for someone who has a broken tooth:

1. Clean the part of the tooth remaining in the mouth and the surrounding area.
2. Take the victim to the dentist or an emergency room as soon as possible.

CHEST WOUNDS

The chest is the upper part of the torso. It is enclosed by the ribs, breastbone, and vertebral

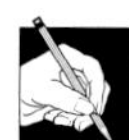

column. It contains the heart, lungs, and diaphragm. Chest wounds can be open or closed. If the wound is open, it is most likely the result of a puncture wound. If the puncture has penetrated the lungs, you will hear a sucking sound coming from the wound with each breath the victim takes. If the person has received a forceful blow to the chest and the wound is closed, you should suspect damage to the ribs or lungs. Use the following steps to care for someone with an open chest wound when the object which caused the wound is still impaled in the body:

1. Call for help.
2. Do not remove the object that caused the wound.
3. Put padding around the object to stabilize it and prevent any movement.
4. Treat for shock.
5. Keep the victim from moving until medical help arrives.
6. Monitor for breathing and circulation.

Use the following steps to care for someone with an open chest wound without an impaled object:

1. Call for help.
2. Cover the wound to prevent outside air from getting into the chest cavity. You can use plastic wrap, a plastic bag, a latex glove, or aluminum foil.
3. Tape the covering down, leaving one corner open so air will not be trapped in the chest cavity.
4. Treat for shock.
5. Keep the victim from moving until medical help arrives.
6. Monitor for breathing and circulation.

Use the following steps to care for someone with a closed chest wound caused by a blow to the chest:

1. Call for help.
2. Have the victim rest comfortably.
3. Have the victim hold a pillow against the injured area.
4. Monitor for internal bleeding.
5. Treat for shock.

STRAINS

Strains usually occur when a muscle is awkwardly stretched too far because of poor lifting position or posture. This action results in a tear to either the muscle fibers or the tendons connecting the muscles to bone. Strains can be caused by lifting a heavy object or working a muscle too hard.

SPRAINS

Sprains occur when a joint is twisted or stretched outside of its normal range of motion. This action results in one or more of the ligaments holding the bones of the joint in place being overstretched, frayed, or torn. The tear can be partial or complete. Sprains most commonly occur in the ankle, knee, wrist, and fingers.

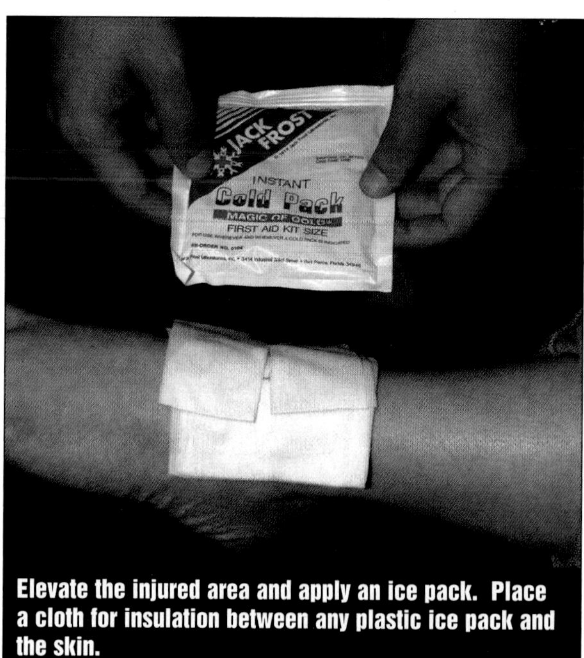

Elevate the injured area and apply an ice pack. Place a cloth for insulation between any plastic ice pack and the skin.

FIRST AID FOR STRAINS AND SPRAINS

Use the following steps to care for a strain, sprain, or bruise:

1. Get the victim into a comfortable, resting position.
2. Elevate the injured area.

3. Apply an ice pack to the injured area. Place a cloth for insulation between any plastic ice pack and the skin.
4. Wrap the injured area with a bandage to hold the ice pack in place. Do not wrap the bandage too tightly.
5. Treat for shock.
6. Transport to medical care, if necessary.

HAND, FINGER, AND FOOT INJURIES

Injuries to the hands, fingers, and feet can occur in the bone, muscle, joints, ligaments, or the nails. See the chapter on soft tissue injuries for more information about cuts and scrapes and their associated first aid. See below for more information about the first aid for fractures and dislocations.

Finger Injuries

Further injuries to the fingers can include:

- Jammed finger. The end of a straightened finger receives a blow. This stretches and tears the ligaments and tendons of the finger.
- Crushed fingertip. The end of a finger is closed in a door or a heavy object falls on the finger. The end of the finger might have a cut, a blood blister, or a bruise. The fingernail might also be damaged.
- Blood under the fingernail (subungual hematoma). The end of the finger is crushed and a blood clot forms under the fingernail.
- Torn nail. The fingernail is caught on an object and tears.

Use the following steps for a jammed finger:

1. Check the range of motion of the finger. Can the victim bend and straighten the finger?
2. Soak the finger in cold water for 20 minutes.
3. Protect the finger by taping it to the next finger if the pain is more than mild.

Use the following steps for a crushed fingertip:

1. Apply an ice pack to the crushed finger for 20 minutes. Place a cloth for insulation between any plastic ice pack and the skin.
2. Wash the finger with soap and water for 5 minutes.
3. Trim any pieces of torn, dead skin with scissors.
4. Cover any cuts with antibiotic ointment and a bandage.

Use the following steps for blood under the fingernail:

1. Apply an ice pack to the finger for 20 minutes.
2. Seek medical treatment if the pain is severe. A physician might drill a hole in the nail to relieve the pressure.

Use the following steps if a fingernail is torn:

1. If the nail is cracked, but does not have any rough edges, leave it alone.
2. Use sterile scissors to cut the torn fingernail along the line of the tear.
3. Apply antibiotic ointment and cover it with a bandage.
4. Change the bandage daily until the nail bed is covered with new skin. A new nail will grow back in six to twelve weeks.

Achilles Tendon Rupture

One further injury to the foot can be an Achilles Tendon rupture. The Achilles Tendon is the strong tendon that joins the calf muscle to the bone of the heel. The signs and symptoms of an Achilles Tendon rupture include:

- Pain in the area above the heel and behind the ankle or up the back of the leg depending on the level the tendon is injured - it often is quite high where the tendon inserts into the calf
- Weakness in the foot
- Inability to flex the foot back toward the shin although victim may be able to weakly extend the foot the other way toward the sole

- Bruising
- Bunching of the calf muscle

Use the following steps if someone has an Achilles Tendon rupture:

1. Get the victim into a comfortable, resting position.
2. Apply an ice pack to the injured area. Place a cloth for insulation between any plastic ice pack and the skin.
3. Wrap the injured area with an elastic bandage to compress the injured area. Do not wrap the bandage too tightly.
4. Elevate the injured area.
5. Treat for shock.
6. Transport to medical care, if necessary.

FRACTURES AND DISLOCATIONS

There are over 200 bones in the human body. Because they are hard and dense (which makes them strong and rigid), they are not easily injured, although injuries still occur. The two types of injuries to bones are fractures and dislocations.

A fracture is a break, chip, or crack in a bone. Fractures can be open (the bone tears through the surface of the skin) or closed. Closed fractures are more common.

A dislocation occurs at a joint. One or more bones move out of their normal position. Dislocations are usually caused by a violent movement, which strains or tears the ligaments holding the bones in place.

Signs and Symptoms

The signs and symptoms of a fracture or dislocation include:

- A deformity of the limb or the limb may be positioned at an odd angle
- Swelling and discoloration
- A grating noise or feeling. The person may have heard an audible popping sound
- Pain
- An inability to move the injured area
- An exposed bone

The general steps for aiding a victim with a fracture or dislocation are:

1. Immobilize the injured area.
2. Apply an ice pack to control swelling and help reduce pain. Place a cloth for insulation between any plastic ice pack and the skin.
3. Call for help or transport the victim to a medical center.
4. Treat for shock.
5. Treat any secondary injuries.
6. Check the pulse at the distal (far) end of a limb, for example, the wrist or foot of an arm or leg injury.

SPLINTING PRINCIPLES AND PRACTICE

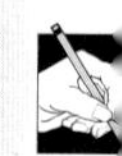

Splinting an injured limb helps to immobilize the area, relieve pain, and protect the limb from further injury. Remember the following points when splinting an injury:

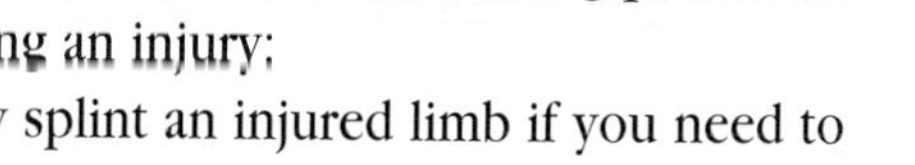

- Only splint an injured limb if you need to move or transport the victim.
- Only splint an injured limb if you can do it without causing further pain and discomfort to the victim.
- Splint the injured limb in the same position in which you found it.
- Splint the injured area as well as the joints above and below the injury. For a dislocation, immobilize the affected joint.
- If a broken bone is exposed, cover the area with a sterile dressing. Do not attempt to reinsert the bone ends.
- Check for adequate circulation below the injured area after you have finished the splint.

You can use many different objects as splints. Splints can be rigid, soft, or anatomic. Some examples of rigid splints are:

- Boards
- Folded newspapers
- Magazines

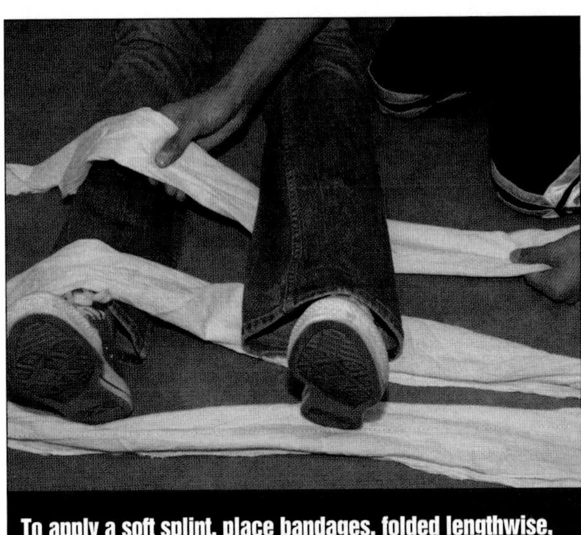
To apply a soft splint, place bandages, folded lengthwise, under the injured area.

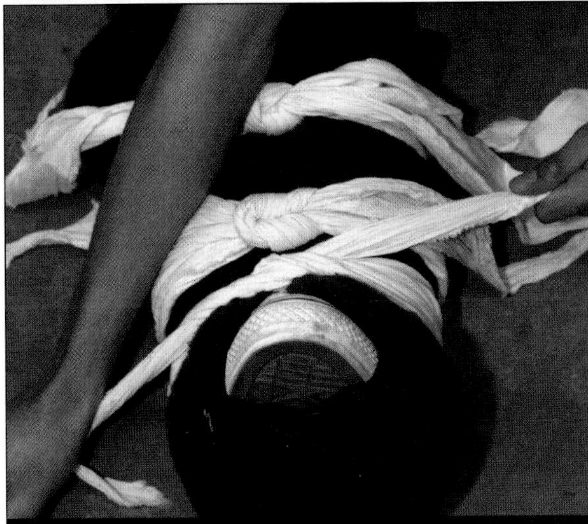
Tie the bandages around the soft splint and the injured area and recheck for pulse feeling, warmth, and color below the site of the injury.

Some examples of soft splints are:

- Folded blankets or towels
- Pillows
- Wetsuits

Some examples of anatomic splints are:

- Taping an injured finger to the finger next to it
- Splinting the injured leg to the uninjured leg

Bandages for splinting can take many forms. Triangular bandages are very common. If triangular

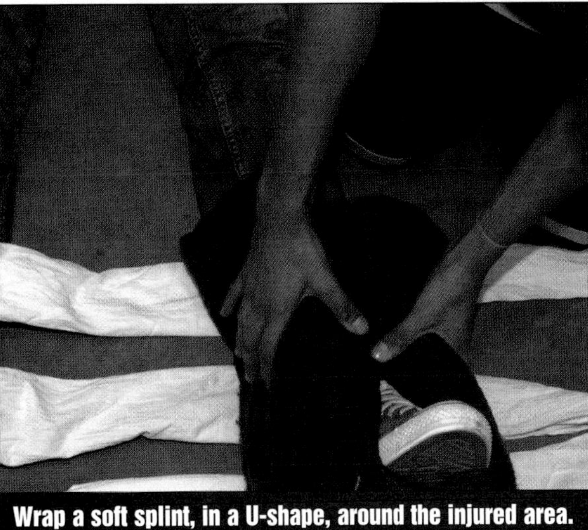
Wrap a soft splint, in a U-shape, around the injured area.

bandages are not available, most any clean bandage of the appropriate size will work. Some examples of bandages are:

- Kerlix®
- ACE™ bandage (elastic bandage)
- Medical tape (2 to 4 inches wide/5 to 8 centimeters wide)

Skill Performance

Use the following steps to apply a rigid splint:

1. Support the injured area and the area above and below the injury. Ask the victim to assist with support if they are able.
2. Check for pulse, feeling, warmth, and color below the site of the injury.
3. Select a rigid splint long enough to immobilize the injured area as well as the joints above and below the injury.
4. Place the rigid splint under the injured area.
   - If splinting a forearm, place a roll of cloth under the palm so that the hand can be comfortably curved
5. Space and tie bandages along the length of the splint to hold it and the broken bones in position.
6. If appropriate, apply a sling or sling and swath for an arm injury to further immobilize the injury.

7. Recheck for feeling, warmth, and color below the site of the injury.

Use the following steps to apply a soft splint:

1. Support the area above and below the injury. Ask the victim to assist with support if they are able.
2. Check for pulse, feeling, warmth, and color below the site of the injury.
3. Select a soft splint large enough to immobilize the injured area as well as the joints above and below the injury.
4. Place bandages, folded lengthwise, under the injured area.
5. Wrap a soft splint, in a U shape, around the injured area.
6. Tie the bandages around the soft splint and the injured area and recheck for pulse feeling, warmth, and color below the site of the injury.

Use the following steps to apply an anatomic splint:

1. Support the area above and below the injury. Ask the victim to assist with support if they are able.
2. Check for pulse, feeling, warmth, and color below the site of the injury.
3. Place bandages, folded lengthwise, under the injured area.
4. Tie the bandages around the injured area and the supporting limb or digit.
5. Recheck for feeling, warmth, and color below the site of the injury.

SPECIAL CONSIDERATIONS FOR CRUSHING INJURIES

Crushing injuries occur when a part of the body is compressed under a force. If the force is applied to a large muscle mass (for example, the thigh area), it can cause Crush Injury Syndrome. When the muscle mass is compressed by the force, it causes several things to occur, including the body to produce large amounts of acid and complex electrolytes (especially potassium) around the affected muscles. Once the force is released, the blood carries the acid and complex electrolytes to the heart. This action can be fatal to the victim. Also, the release of the force can cause a sudden loss of blood.

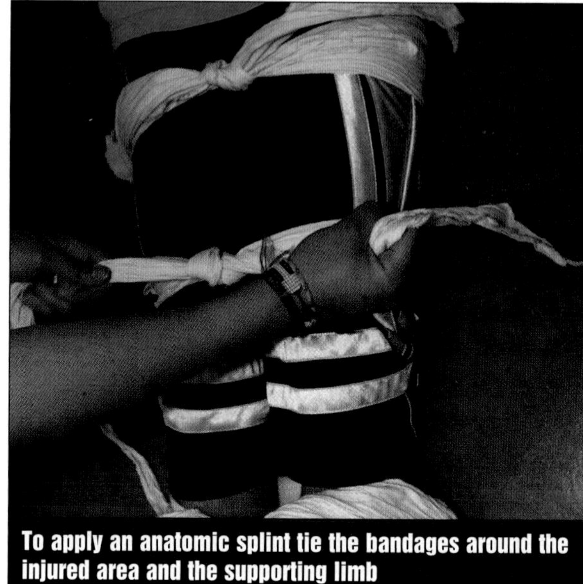

To apply an anatomic splint tie the bandages around the injured area and the supporting limb

You must be aware of this syndrome and consider it as a potential problem when the following criteria are seen:

- Involvement of a large muscle mass
- Prolonged compression
- Compromised blood circulation

For example, an entrapped hand is not likely to cause the syndrome. The signs and symptoms of Crush Injury Syndrome are:

- Compression of a large muscle mass
- Compression of the muscle mass for longer than 60 minutes
- No pulse or capillary return in the limb beyond the compression site
- Pale, cool, and clammy skin
- Weak and rapid pulse
- Absence of pain in the affected region
- Symptoms and signs of shock

Use the following steps if you see a compression injury:

1. Call for help.
2. If the muscle mass has been compressed for less then 60 minutes, remove the crushing force as quickly and gently as possible, if it is safe to do so. If it has been more than 60 minutes, wait for help to arrive.

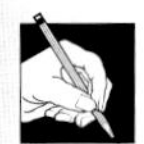

3. Treat any other injuries.
4. Treat for shock.
5. Reassure the victim.

REVIEW QUESTIONS

1. There are two types of head injuries: ______________________________

2. Signs and symptoms of a head injury include: - list 5 of 9 symptoms from the text.

____

____

____

____

____

3. You should always suspect a neck, or spinal injury in any of the following situations: - list 6 of 10 situations from the text.

____

____

____

____

____

____

4. Use the following steps to care for someone who has had a tooth knocked out: - list 3 of the 4 steps from the text. ______________________________

____

____

5. Chest wounds can be ______________________________ .

6. Strains usually occur when a muscle is ____________________ because of _______

____

7. Sprains occur when a ____ outside of its normal range of motion.

8. The signs and symptoms of a fracture or dislocation include: - list 4 of 6 signs or symptoms from the text.____

   ____

   ____

   ____

9. Splinting an injured limb helps to ____

   ____

10. If the muscle mass has been compressed for less then _______________, remove the crushing force as quickly and gently as possible, if it is safe to do so. If it has been more than _______________, wait for help to arrive.

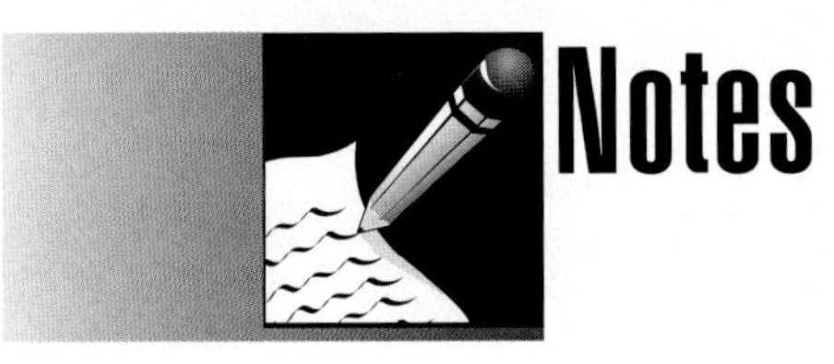

Notes

CHAPTER 13

Poisoning, Stings, and Bites

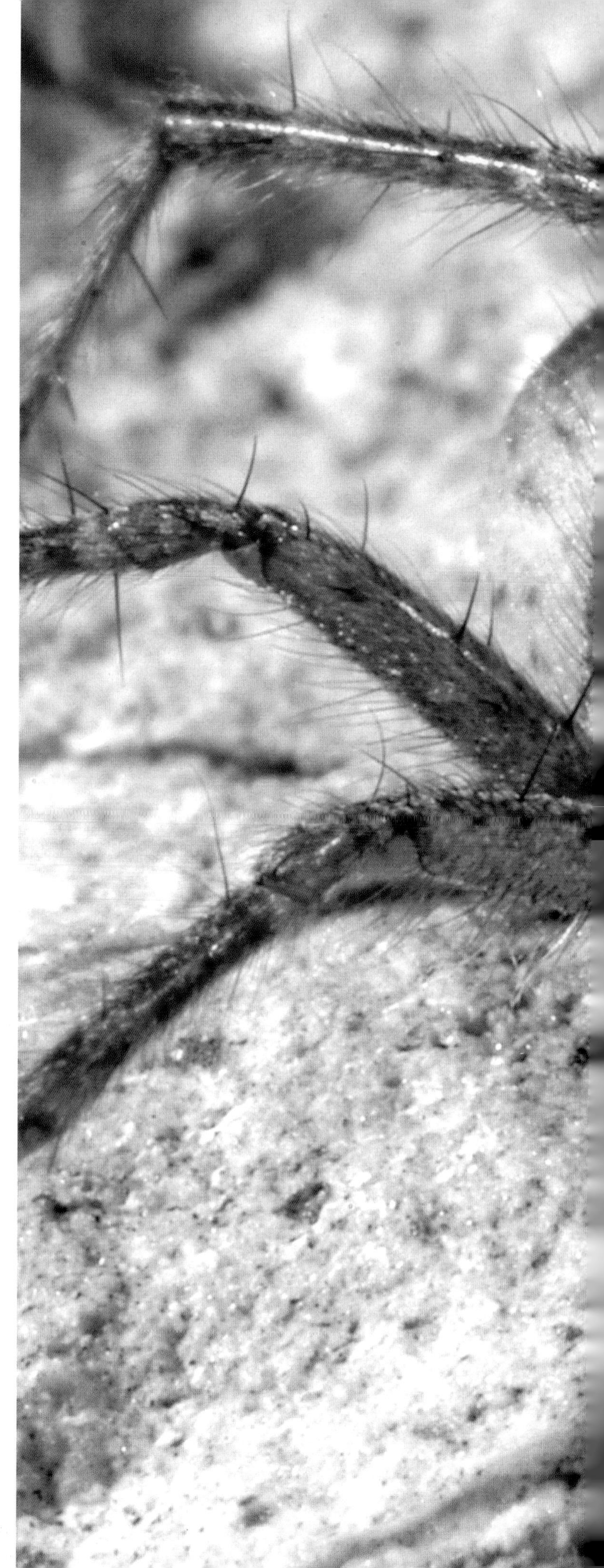

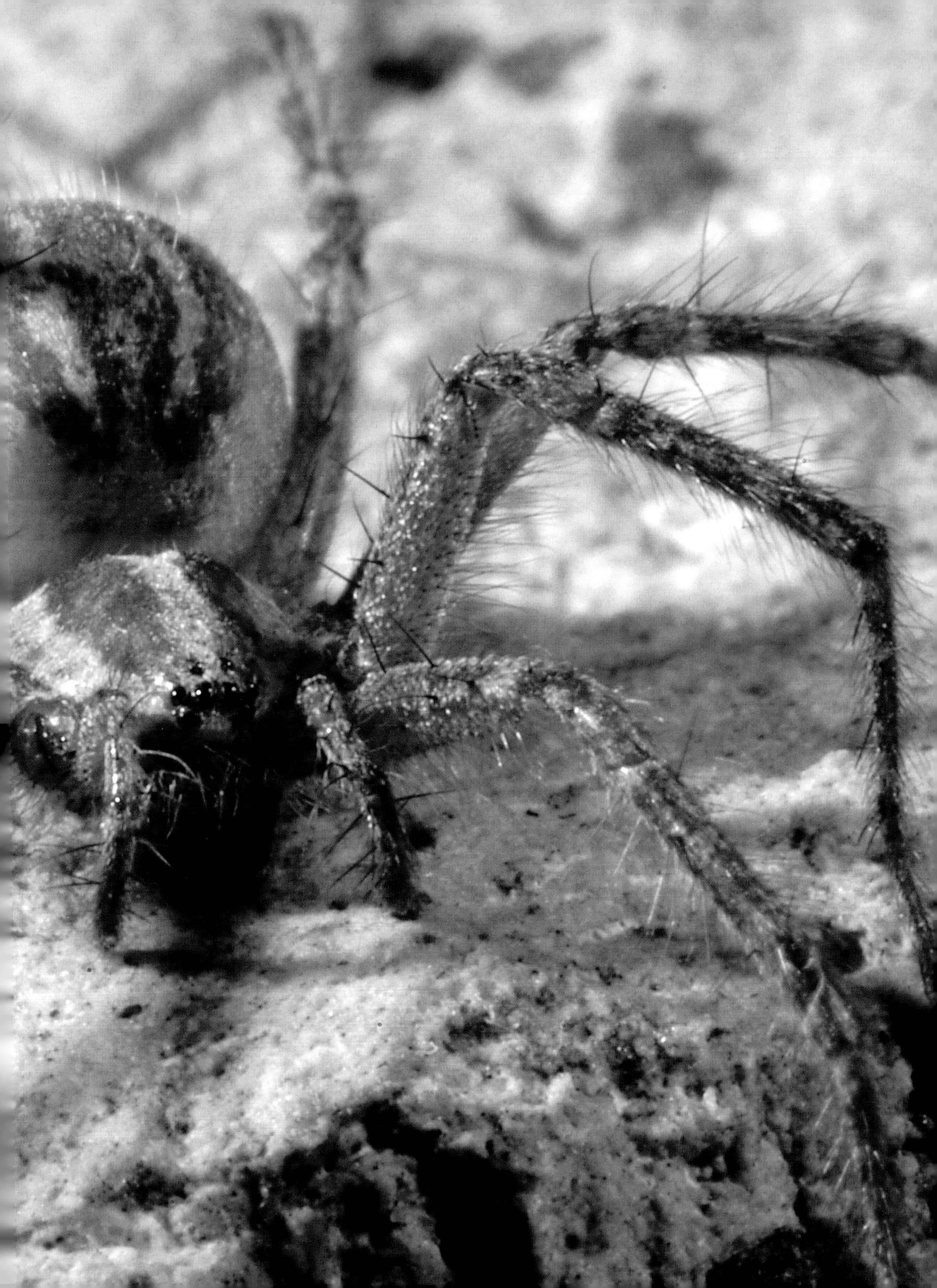

There are some injuries that require special procedures for first aid.

LEARNING GOALS

In this chapter you will learn about:

- Poisoning
- Insect bites and stings
- Animal bites and envenomations

POISONS

Poisons are substances (usually chemical in nature) that cause injury, illness, or death, especially by chemical means that can cause tissue or organ damage.

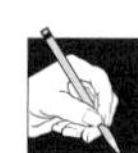

Poisons can be in liquid, solid, or gaseous form. They can be swallowed, injected, inhaled, or absorbed into the body. They can negatively affect your health and can even cause death.

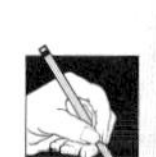

When you suspect that a person has been poisoned, call the Poison Control Center immediately. Be prepared to tell them what type of poison and how much was involved. They will direct you in how to provide appropriate first aid. Many countries throughout the world maintain their own Poison Control Centers. When you travel to a foreign country, check the internet for the number of their Poison Control Center and make it a part of your first aid kit. One source for finding a U.S. or international Poison Control Center is the World Health Organization (WHO) http://www.who.int. In the United States, the national poison control emergency number is 1-800-222-1222. If you call this number, they will connect you directly to your own state's Poison Control Center.

Also see "Marine Life Injuries" in chapter 18 for further information on first aid for marine life envenomations and ingested fish poisoning.

INGESTED POISONS

Ingested poisons are substances that a person swallows. Ingested poisons can include foods such as mushrooms and shellfish, alcohol, medications, household and garden items, and some plants. You can prevent accidental ingestion of poisons by:

- Keeping all medicines, household and garden items, cleaning products, and poisonous plants out of reach or under lock and key.
- Keeping all medicines, including travel medicines, in the original bottles.
- Following directions on medications for proper dosages.
- Don't take medicine in the dark.
- Disposing of any unused medicines.
- Storing harmful substances away from food.
- Keeping poisonous substances in their original packaging.

General Symptoms

Someone who has ingested a poison might have some of the following signs and symptoms:

- Abdominal cramping or pain
- Nausea and possibly vomiting
- Diarrhea
- Burns, stains, or an odor in or around their mouth
- Changes in consciousness

Care

Use the following steps if you suspect someone has ingested a poison:

1. Assess the scene for safety and to determine the type of poisoning.
2. Perform a primary assessment of the victim.
3. Provide care for any life-threatening conditions.
4. Ask the victim, if they are conscious, what they ate.
5. Call the Poison Control Center or your local emergency number.

INHALED POISONS

Inhaled poisons are substances that a victim breathes into their lungs through either the nose or mouth. Inhaled poisons can include exhaust from incomplete combustion in an engine, automobile, or home heating system (carbon monoxide), sulfur dioxide from wells and sewers, chlorine gas from swimming pools, and fumes from paints, glues, and cleaners.

General Symptoms

Someone who has inhaled a poison might have some of the following signs and symptoms:

- Pale or bluish colored skin
- Nausea and possibly vomiting
- Breathing difficulties
- Changes in consciousness
- Seizures

Care

Use the following steps if you suspect someone has inhaled a poison:

1. Assess the scene for safety.
2. Remove the victim from the area if the fumes are still present. Be sure to protect yourself from inhaling the fumes.
3. Perform a primary assessment of the victim.
4. Provide care for any life-threatening conditions.
5. Ask the victim, if they are conscious, what they inhaled.
6. Call the Poison Control Center or your local emergency number.
7. If carbon monoxide poisoning is suspected provide oxygen first aid and arrange emergency transport to a medical facility.

CONTACT POISONS

Contact poisons are absorbed through the skin. Poisonous plants such as poison ivy, poison oak,

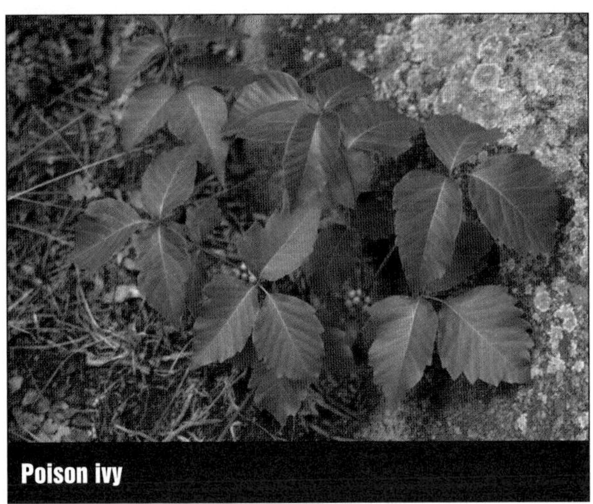
Poison ivy

poisonwood, or poison sumac, fertilizers, solvents, and pesticides are examples of contact poisons.

General Symptoms

Someone who has come in contact with a poisonous plant or substance might have the following signs and symptoms:

- Skin irritation
- Itching
- Weeping sores

Care

Use the following steps if you think someone has come in contact with a poisonous plant or substance:

1. Immediately wash the affected area with soap and water.
2. If weeping sores develop, apply calamine lotion to the affected area.

Anti-inflammatory drugs (such as corticosteroids) or Benedryl™ can help relieve discomfort.

BITES AND STINGS

There are many species of insects that can sting or bite you. Usually the stings are not dangerous. However, some people can have severe allergic reactions to stings. You can also be bitten by a snake or a household pet.

Stings from Bees, Wasps, Hornets, and Scorpions

Bees, wasps, hornets, and scorpions inject venom through the skin of their victim. Only the honeybee embeds its stinger in the victim and leaves it there, killing the bee. Hornets, wasps, scorpions and other insects inject their poison and can continue to sting repeatedly. The symptoms of a sting from a bee, wasp, hornet, or scorpion are:

- Pain around the affected area
- Swelling around the affected area
- Stinger with poison sac embedded in the skin (honeybees only)

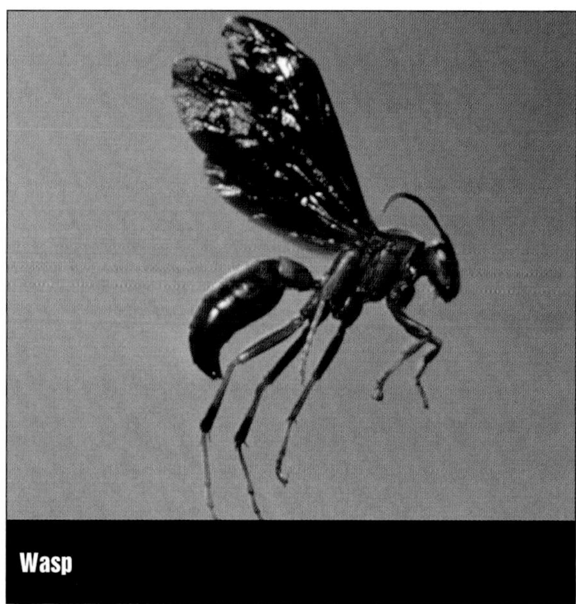
Wasp

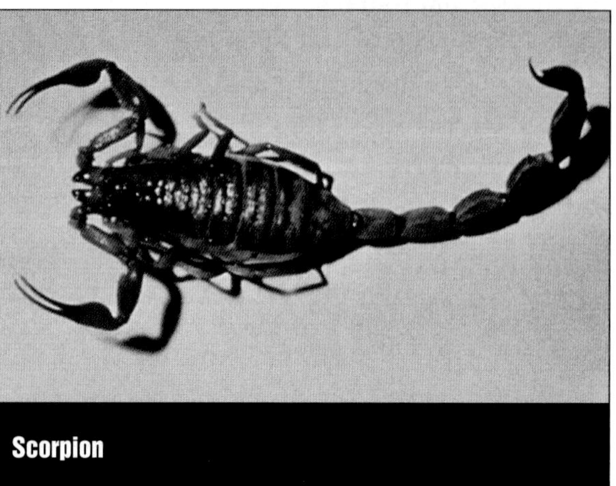
Scorpion

The steps to care for a sting from a bee, wasp, hornet, or scorpion are:

1. For a bee sting, remove the stinger as quickly as possible. A bee's stinger should be scraped out using a fingernail, knife blade, or plastic card. *Do not remove the stinger by grabbing it with your fingers or by using tweezers to pull it out. The poison sac is still attached to the stinger and will inject more poison.*
2. Wash the area thoroughly.
3. Apply a cold pack to the affected area.
4. Monitor the victim for signs of an allergic reaction. (See "Severe Allergic Reactions" in Chapter 15 for further information on allergic reactions.)

Bites from Spiders

There are a few species of spiders that are considered harmful and potentially deadly. They include (among others):

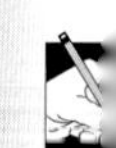

- The black widow spider (North America) and the related button spider (southern Africa).
- The brown recluse spider (North America).
- The funnel-web spider (Australia).

The Black Widow Spider

The black widow spider is shiny black with a red hourglass mark on the underside of its body.

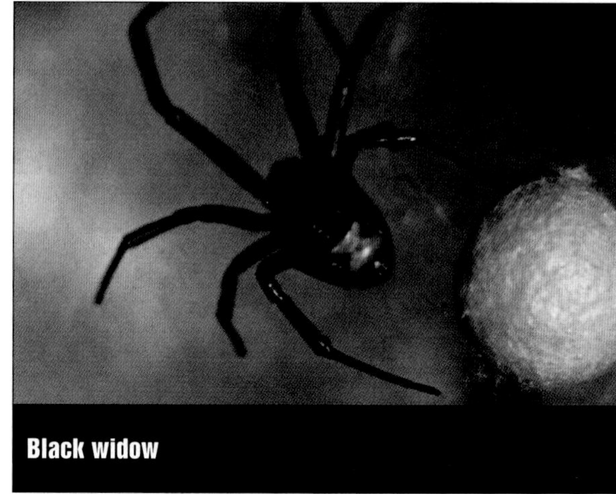
Black widow

They spin a sticky, irregular web and prefer dark, quiet areas such as garages or wood piles. Black widow spider bites inject a neurotoxin and can be deadly to children and older adults, but are rarely fatal for healthy adults. The signs and symptoms of a bite from a black widow spider include:

- Pain around the affected area that starts one to three hours after the bite and can last up to 48 hours.
- Swelling around the affected area.
- Nausea and vomiting.
- Difficulty breathing or swallowing.

The steps to care for a bite are:

1. Wash the area thoroughly.
2. Apply a cold pack to the affected area.
3. Call for help or transport the victim to medical care.
4. Monitor the victim for signs of an allergic reaction. (See Chapter 15, "Severe Allergic Reactions" for further information on allergic reactions.)

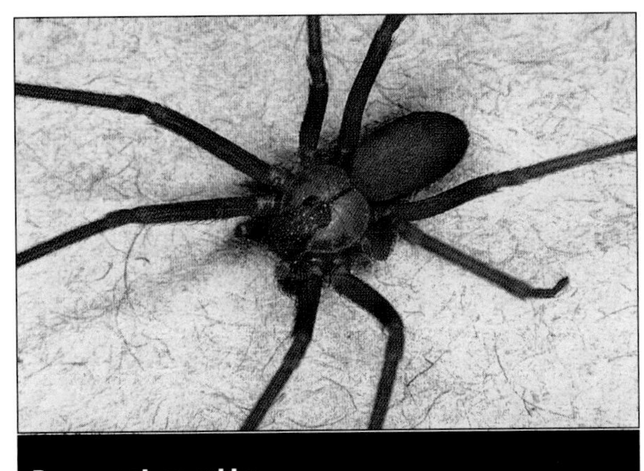

Brown recluse spider

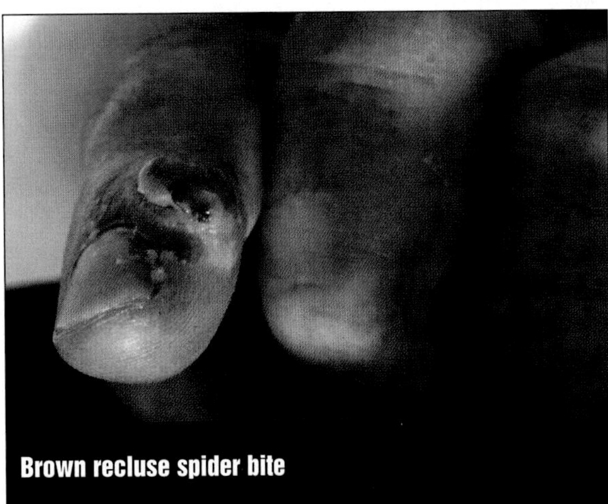

Brown recluse spider bite

The Brown Recluse Spider

The brown recluse spider is a yellowish to brown color and violin shaped. They hide in wood, rock, or brush piles or other dark places. (Most likely found in the Southeast US, and a lesser toxic species exists in the Western US). Brown recluse spider bites inject a local toxin and cause serious tissue destruction, but severe (fatal) systemic reactions are extremely rare. The signs and symptoms of a bite from a brown recluse spider include:

- The feeling of being stung followed by intense pain
- A wound that looks like a red or purplish blister, or black necrotic spot surrounded by a reddish discoloration and swelling with a "bull's-eye" appearance

The steps to care for a bite are:

1. Wash the area thoroughly.
2. Apply a cold pack to the affected area.
3. Call for help or transport the victim to medical care.
4. Monitor the victim for signs of an allergic reaction. (See Chapter 15, "Severe Allergic Reactions" for further information on allergic reactions.)

The Funnel-Web Spider

The funnel-web spider is found in eastern Australia in coastal and highland forest regions. It is a large spider (0.5 - 2 inches/1.5 - 4.5 cm) that is a dark brown to black color with a dark plum to black abdomen. They burrow in moist, cool, sheltered habitats, such as under rocks or in or under rotting logs. Funnel-web spider bites inject a neurotoxin and cause serious illness or death.

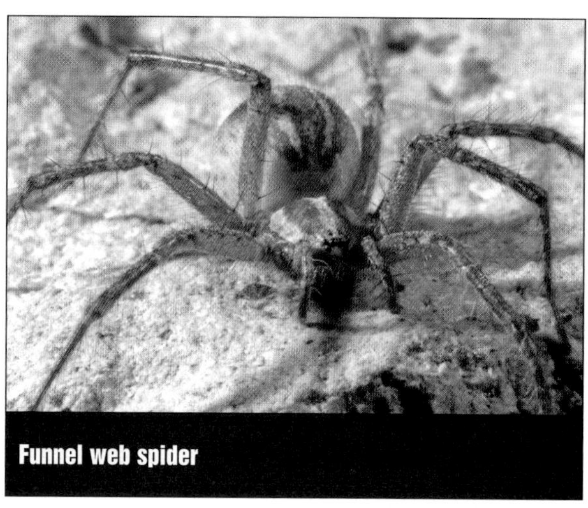

Funnel web spider

The signs and symptoms of a bite from a funnel-web spider include:

- Pain in the area of the bite
- Mouth numbness
- Vomiting
- Abdominal pain
- Sweating and salivation

The steps to care for a bite are:

1. Place a cloth or gauze pad that measures four inches by four inches (10 cm by 10 cm) by an inch (2.5 cm) thick directly over the wound. Do not wash off any venom.
2. Hold the pad in place by wrapping an elastic bandage around the pad and the limb. Wrap at least an inch (2.5 cm) above and below the pad. Wrapping the entire limb is better. Wrap the pad tight enough to press the pad into the skin, but not tight enough to cut off circulation.
3. Apply a splint to immobilize the limb.
4. Restrict the victim's movement.
5. Capture the spider for positive identification.
6. Call for help or transport the victim to medical care.

Tick Bites

Ticks live in wooded and grassy areas throughout the world. Common dog and wood ticks are about an eighth of an inch (3 mm) long. Ticks can carry and transmit a wide variety of diseases, including Rocky Mountain spotted fever and Colorado tick fever. Deer ticks, which can transmit Lyme disease, are about the size of the head of a pin. Ticks will attach to any warm-blooded animal that brushes by the tick. Use the following steps if you see a tick attached to someone:

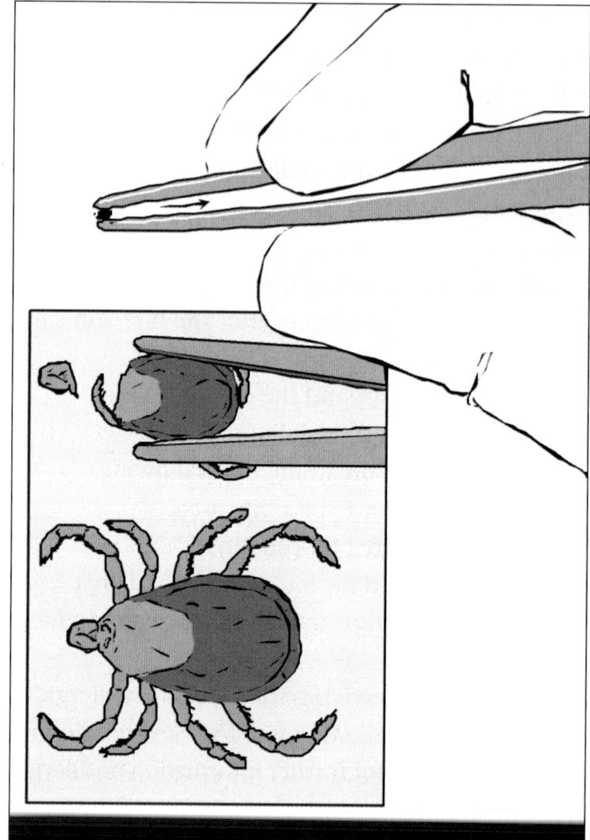

Proper tick removal

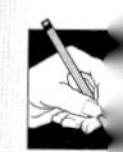

1. Remove the tick with tweezers. Carefully grasp the tick as close to the skin as possible and pull it straight out with a slow, steady pull. Be careful not to squeeze the tick's body, and double check that you got it all.
2. Wash the area with soap and water.
3. Apply an antiseptic ointment.
4. Seek medical attention if you cannot remove the entire tick or if a rash develops.

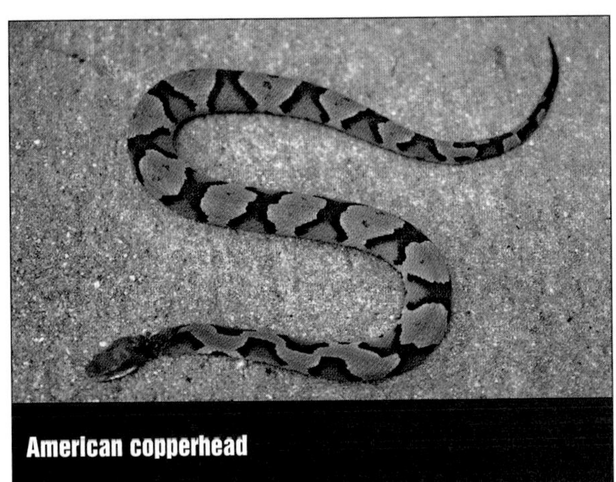
American copperhead

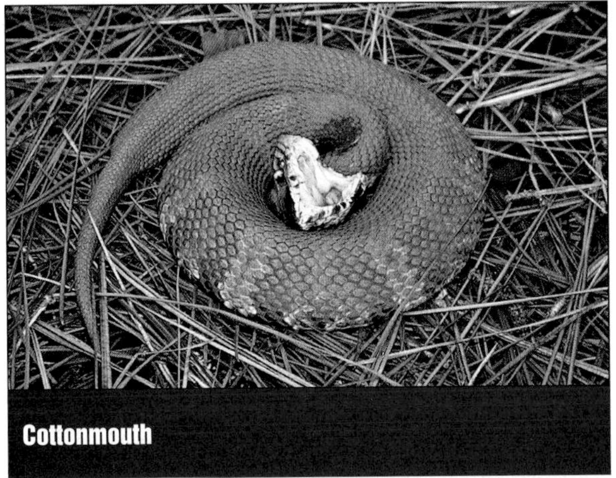
Cottonmouth

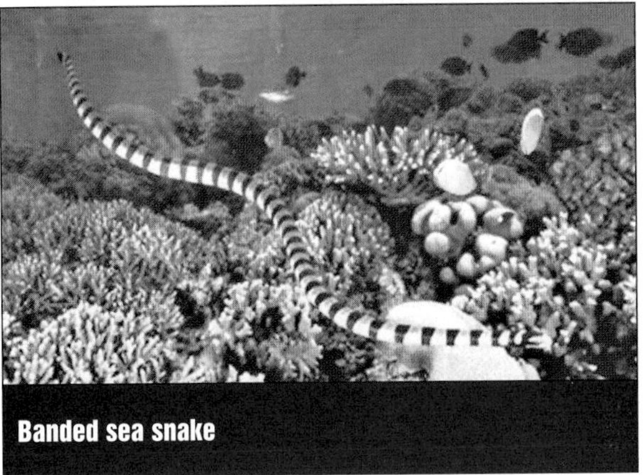
Banded sea snake

Lyme disease is transmitted by the deer tick. The signs and symptoms of Lyme disease include:

- A rash, up to seven inches (18 cm) across in the area of the bite. The rash might have a bull's eye appearance.
- Fever
- Headache
- Weakness
- Joint and muscle pain

Lyme disease is treated with antibiotics. These are most effective when taken early in the disease. If you suspect that someone has Lyme disease, seek medical attention as soon as possible.

Bites from Snakes

Generally, snakes are shy creatures that prefer to be left alone. They will only attack when they feel threatened. There are many types of poisonous snakes throughout the world. Poisonous snakes in North and South America are:

- American copperhead
- Bushmaster
- Coral snake
- Cottonmouth
- Eastern diamondback rattlesnake
- Eyelash pit viper
- Fer-de-lance
- Jumping viper
- Mojave rattlesnake
- Tropical rattlesnake
- Western diamondback rattlesnake

The poisonous snakes in Europe are:

- Common adder
- Long-nosed adder
- Pallas' viper
- Ursini's viper

The poisonous snakes in Africa and Asia are:

- Boomslang
- Bush viper
- Common cobra
- Egyptian cobra
- Gaboon viper
- Green mamba
- Green tree pit viper
- Habu pit viper
- Horned desert viper
- King cobra
- Krait
- Levant viper

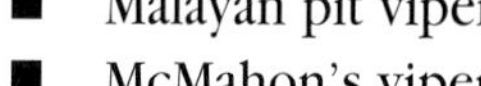

- Malayan pit viper
- McMahon's viper
- Mole viper or burrowing viper
- Palestinian viper
- Puff adder
- Rhinoceros viper or river jack
- Russell's viper
- Sand viper
- Saw-scaled viper
- Wagler's pit viper or temple viper

The poisonous snakes in Australasia are:

- Australian copperhead
- Death adder
- Taipan
- Tiger snake

The poisonous sea snakes are:

- Banded sea snake
- Yellow-bellied sea snake

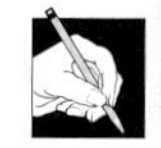

Fully half of all venomous snake bites are without any envenomation or "dry bites." Coral snakes and sea snakes lack the long fangs of the other poisonous snakes and have small mouths, requiring them to chew on something small, such as a finger, in order to inject their venom.

The signs and symptoms of a snake bite include:

- Bite marks
- Pain around the affected area
- Swelling around the affected area

The steps to care for a snake bite are:

1. Wash the area thoroughly.
2. Remove jewelry or tight fitting clothing around the wound.
3. Immobilize the affected area and keep it below the level of the victim's heart.
4. Pressure immobilization is recommended for bites from snakes belonging to the family Elapidae, which includes cobra, coral snake, death adder, krait, mamba, taipan, tiger, and sea snake. The pressure is achieved by applying a snug fitting bandage that will allow you to slip a finger beneath it.
5. Call for help or transport the victim to medical care.

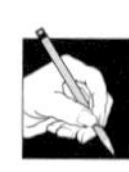

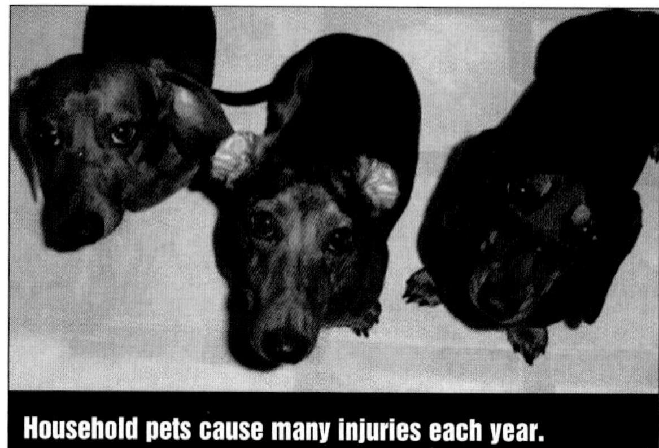

Household pets cause many injuries each year.

Animal Bites

Animal or human bites can cause infection and soft tissue injuries. If the animal that bit the victim is rabid, the bite can also cause rabies. A wild animal that is acting strangely could be rabid. Rabies is virtually 100% fatal if left untreated and once symptoms develop. Use the following steps if someone is bit by an animal and the bite is minor:

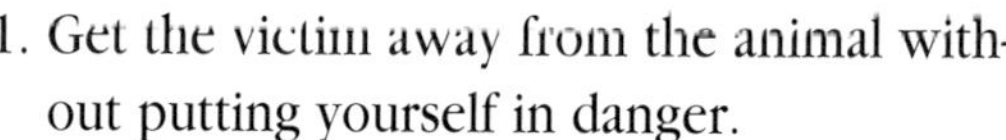

1. Get the victim away from the animal without putting yourself in danger.
2. Control any bleeding.
3. Wash the wound thoroughly with soap and water.
4. Apply an antibiotic ointment and a dressing.
5. Be prepared to treat the victim for shock.
6. Seek medical attention, especially if it is suspected that the animal might have rabies

Use the following steps if someone is bit by an animal and the bite is major:

1. Get the victim away from the animal without putting yourself in danger.
2. Control any bleeding.
3. Be prepared to treat the victim for shock.
4. Seek medical attention or call for help.

Remember as much as possible about the locale in which the bite occurred and what the animal looked like. Do not try to trap the animal yourself. Call the authorities and they will dispatch the appropriate people to look for and catch the animal.

REVIEW QUESTIONS

1. Poisons can be ______________________________. They can be ______________________________ into the body.

2. When you suspect that a person has been poisoned, ______________________.

3. Hornets, wasps, scorpions and other insects inject their poison and ______________.

4. There are a few species of spiders that are considered harmful and potentially deadly. They include (among others): - list 3 of 4 from the text.

   ____

   ____

   ____

5. Generally, snakes are ______________ that prefer ______________. They will only ______________________________.

6. Fully half of all venomous snake bites are ______________________.

7. Pressure immobilization is recommended for bites from snakes belonging to the family Elapidae, which includes ______________________________.

8. Rabies is ______________ if left untreated and once symptoms develop.

9. Ticks can carry and transmit a wide variety of diseases, including ______________.

CHAPTER 14

Other Medical Emergencies

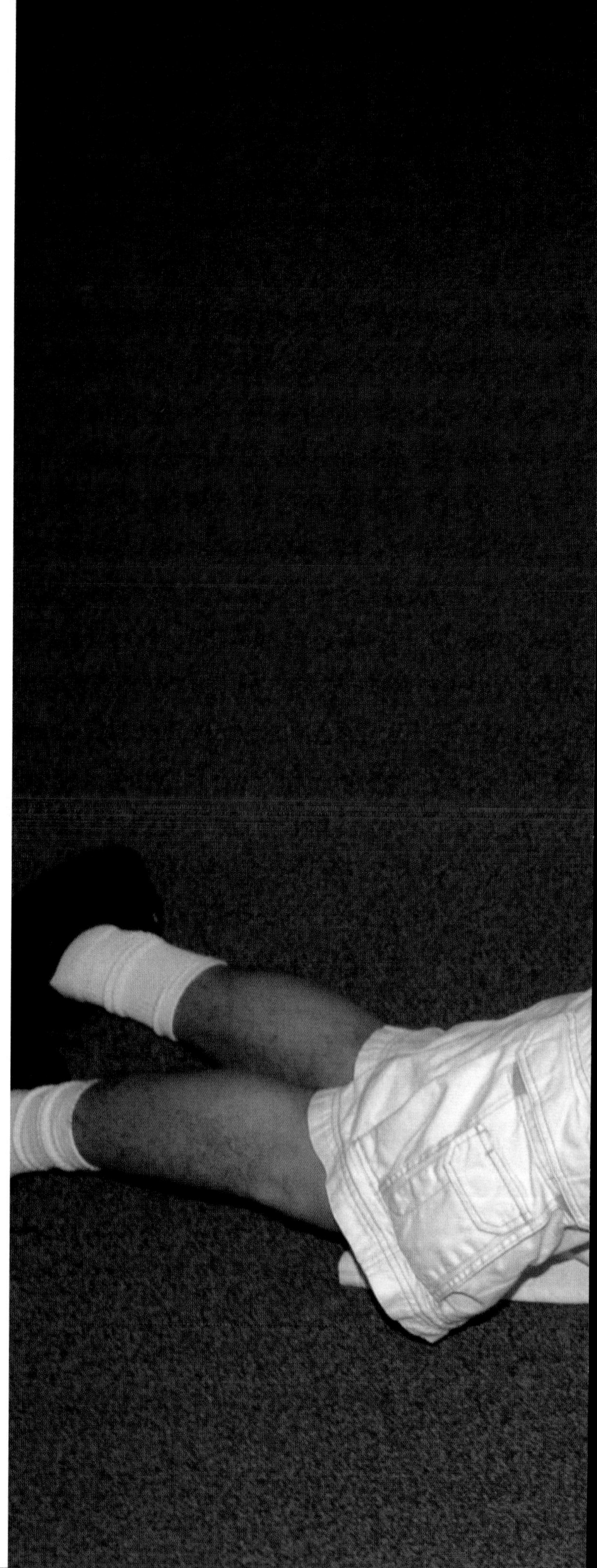

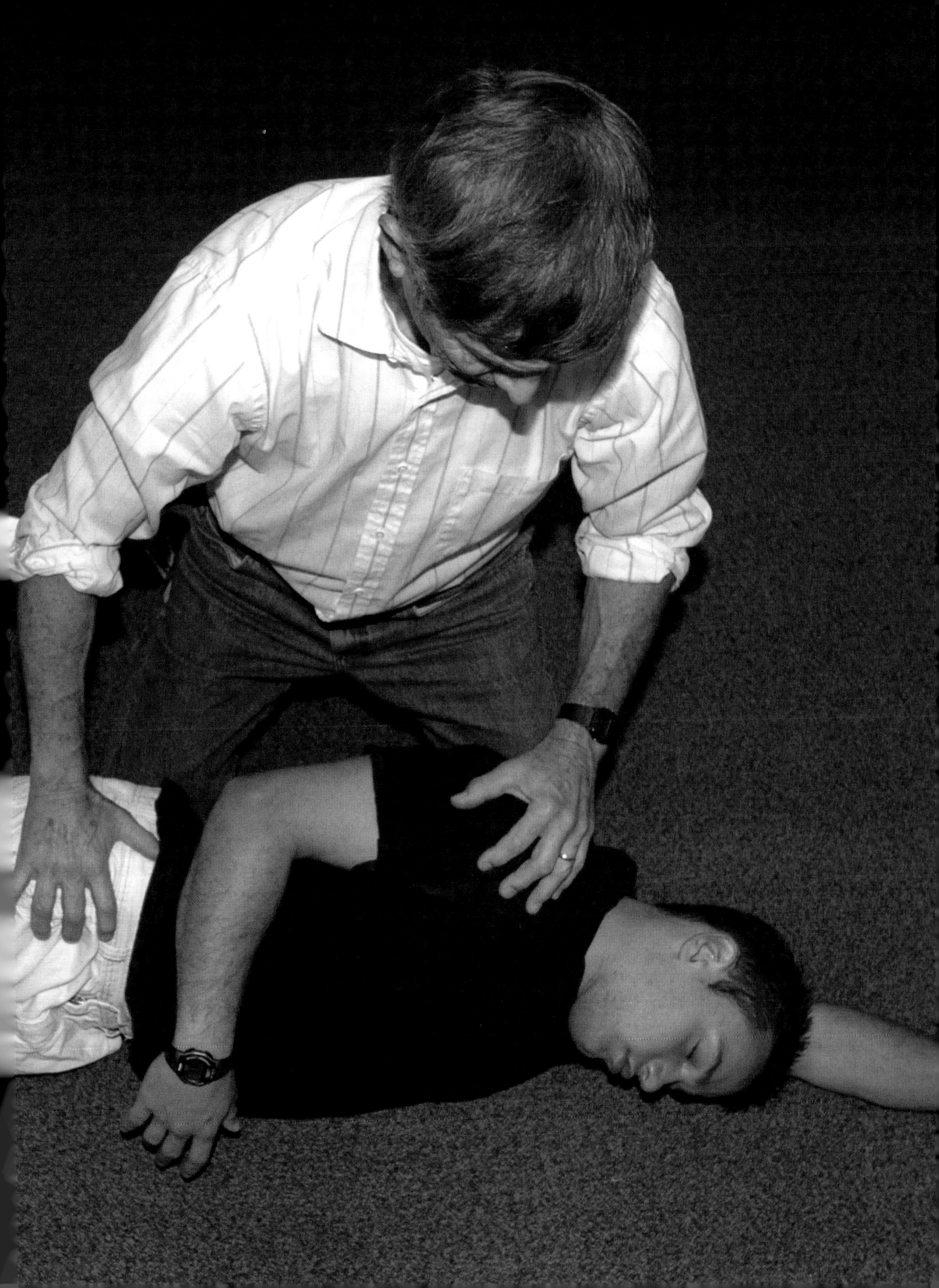

There are many different kinds of medical emergencies. You might not know what the problem is, so you should treat the symptoms and call for help.

LEARNING GOALS

In this chapter you will learn about:

- Fainting
- Asthma and COPD
- Diabetic emergencies
- Epilepsy and seizures
- Anaphylaxis / severe allergic reactions
- Injuries during pregnancy and associated concerns (abdominal injuries, vaginal bleeding, etc.)

The common signs and symptoms of sudden illness include:

- Lightheadedness, dizziness, confusion, or weakness
- Changes in skin color and sweating
- Nausea or vomiting
- Diarrhea

There are also signs and symptoms specific to each type of sudden illness, which will be detailed in each following section. Use the following general steps to deal with a sudden illness:

1. Move the victim to a comfortable position.
2. Interview the victim or bystanders for information. Ask the victim the following questions:
   a. Are you allergic to anything?
   b. Are you taking any medications?
   c. When did you last eat?
   d. What led up to this problem?
3. Look for medical alert tags.
4. Look for changes in breathing and consciousness.
5. Keep the victim from getting chilled or overheated.
6. Call for help, if necessary.

FAINTING

When someone suddenly loses consciousness, they might have simply fainted. There are many causes, but most are associated with decreased blood flow to the brain. Fainting is not usually harmful and the victim quickly recovers. A person who is about to faint usually becomes very pale, begins to sweat profusely and then loses consciousness and collapses.

Use the following steps if someone faints:

1. If you are in a position to prevent their falling, lower a victim to the ground or other flat surface.
2. Position the victim on their back.
3. Raise their legs 8 to 12 inches (20 - 30 cm).
4. Loosen any tight clothing.
5. Check for airway, breathing, and circulation.
6. Check for any injuries suffered during their fall.
7. If the victim vomits or is nauseous, place them on their side in the recovery position.
8. If the victim does not regain consciousness or recover quickly, call for help.

ASTHMA

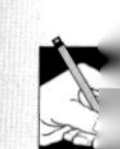

Asthma is a chronic lung disorder that is marked by recurring episodes of airway obstruction. An asthma attack is triggered by hyper-reactivity to any of various stimuli, such as allergens or even a sudden change in air pressure. People with asthma can have reactions to a swallowed substance (medications or foods), an inhaled substance (pollen or pollutants), or an injected substance (an insect sting). Strenuous exercise or stress can also trigger an asthma attack. Asthma is more common in children and young adults. The signs and symptoms of an asthma attack include:

- Wheezing or other strident sound when attempting to breathe
- Difficulty breathing
- Increased pulse rate
- Anxiety

- Distended and bulging neck veins
- Coughing

Use the following steps if someone is having an asthma attack:

1. Help the victim rest comfortably.
2. Assist the victim with their asthma medication, if necessary. Usually people with asthma will carry medication with them.
3. Call for help if the symptoms do not improve or seem to be getting worse.

CHRONIC OBSTRUCTIVE PULMONARY DISEASE

Chronic obstructive pulmonary disease (COPD) refers to any of several diseases of the lungs that are primarily caused by long-term insult to the lungs. Cigarette smoking is a major cause of COPD. The result is a blocking of the airways or reduced elasticity of the lungs, and it has no cure. COPD is permanent. The most common form of COPD is a combination of chronic bronchitis and emphysema.

Chronic bronchitis occurs when the airways in the lungs have become narrow and partly clogged with mucus. The signs and symptoms of chronic bronchitis include:

- Shortness of breath
- Coughing and excessive amounts of sputum
- Wheezing
- Fluid build-up (commonly swelling at the ankles) and a bluish appearance to the skin

Emphysema occurs when some of the alveoli (air sacs) deep in the lungs have been damaged by becoming enlarged or being destroyed. This loss of elasticity also causes the surrounding airways to collapse. The signs and symptoms of emphysema include:

- Shortness of breath from moderate exertion
- Barrel-shaped chest

Use the following steps if someone is having trouble breathing from COPD:

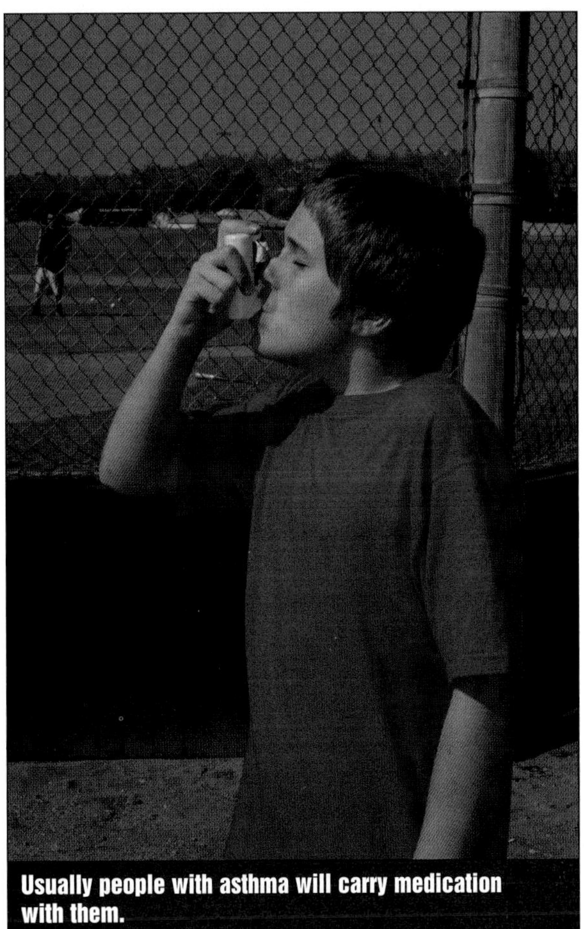

Usually people with asthma will carry medication with them.

1. Calm and reassure the victim.
2. Assist the victim with their prescribed medication, if necessary.
3. Monitor their vital signs.
4. Call for help in the following situations:
   - Any shortness of breath with chest pain.
   - If the victim's symptoms do not improve or seem to be getting worse.
   - If the victim is breathing pure oxygen as part of their treatment regimen.

DIABETIC EMERGENCIES

Diabetes is the inability of the body to convert sugar from food to energy. Some of the symptoms of a diabetic emergency are the same as for other medical emergencies. Diabetics often wear medical alert bracelets or tags signaling their condition.

People who are diabetic can become ill when there is too little or too much sugar in their bloodstream. If a diabetic's blood sugar is too low (hypoglycemia), their signs and symptoms can include:

- Shakiness
- Dizziness
- Sweating
- Hunger
- Headache
- Paleness
- Sudden moodiness or behavior changes for no reason
- Clumsiness
- Seizures
- Confusion
- Unconsciousness

If a diabetic's blood sugar is too high (hyperglycemia), their signs and symptoms can include:

- High blood sugar, which can only be determined by a blood test
- Sugar in the urine, which can only be determined by a urine test
- Frequent urination
- Increased thirst
- Ketoacidosis, which is a buildup of ketone bodies in the bloodstream that can present the following signs and symptoms:
  - Fruity-smelling breath
  - Shortness of breath
  - Nausea and vomiting
  - Dry mouth

Use the following steps if someone is having a diabetic emergency and is conscious:

1. Ask the victim if they have diabetes.
2. Ask them when they ate last.
3. Give the victim some type of sugar (soft drink, candy bar, refined sugar, or honey are some examples). If the victim's problem is high blood sugar, giving the victim sugar will not adversely affect them. If the problem is hypoglycemia, giving them sugar will reduce or terminate the symptoms.

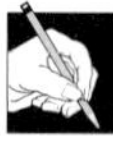

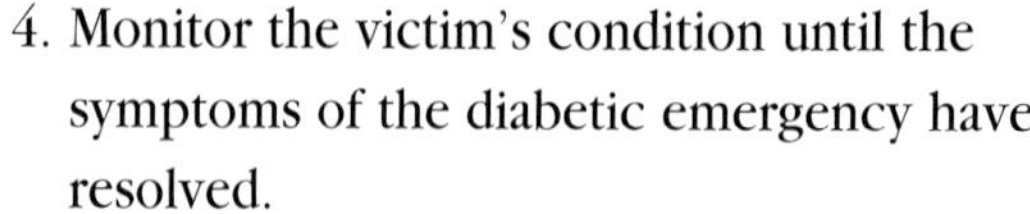

4. Monitor the victim's condition until the symptoms of the diabetic emergency have resolved.
5. Call for help if the symptoms do not improve after administering sugar.

Use the following steps if someone is having a diabetic emergency and is unconscious:

1. Check for a medical alert tag.
2. Call for help.

SEIZURES AND EPILEPSY

Seizures occur when the electrical activity of the brain becomes irregular. This irregular activity can be due to disease, fever, infection, or an injury to the brain. Seizures can also be a result of a medical condition known as epilepsy. Seizures can range from apparent loss of awareness to blackouts to sudden and severe convulsions. Usually the seizures last only a few minutes and the person recovers without experiencing any residual problems. Following a seizure a victim might be confused for a few minutes to an hour. Use the following steps if someone is having a seizure:

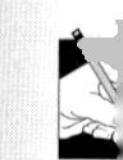

1. Clear the area of any objects that can harm the victim.
2. Do not hold or restrain the victim.
3. Do not try to place anything in the victim's mouth.
4. Cushion the victim's head.
5. Place the victim on their side in the recovery position when the seizure stops to prevent choking.
6. When the victim regains consciousness, determine if they are taking prescribed anticonvulsants, and if so encourage them to take their medication as soon as possible.
7. Call for help in any of the following situations:
   - You do not know the cause of the seizure

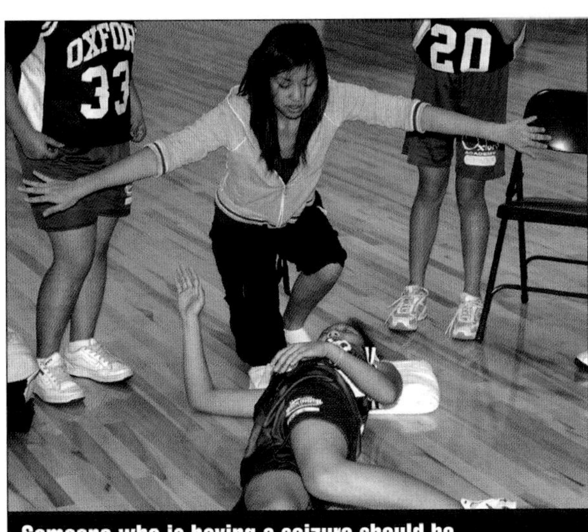

Someone who is having a seizure should be protected from harm but must not be restrained.

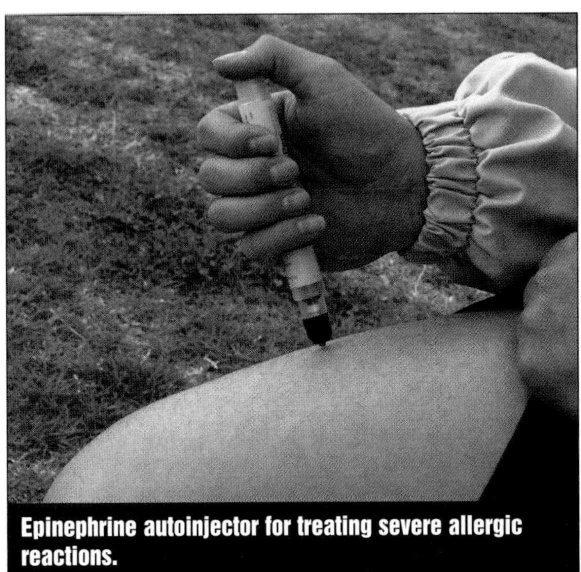

Epinephrine autoinjector for treating severe allergic reactions.

- The seizure lasts for more than three minutes or the victim has multiple seizures
- The victim is pregnant
- The victim does not regain consciousness
- The victim is injured
- The seizure occurs in the water

Children can sometimes have seizures due to a high fever. This is a medical emergency. The fever needs to be reduced and the child needs medical attention.

SEVERE ALLERGIC REACTIONS

Severe allergic reactions or anaphylactic shock are life-threatening conditions and require medical attention. If they are not treated, they can be fatal. The reaction is a result of a person encountering a substance to which they are extremely allergic. These substances can be:

- Ingested, such as nuts, fish, shellfish, spices, or medications
- Inhaled, such as dust, pollen, or chemicals
- Absorbed, such as chemicals
- Injected, such as antitoxins, drugs, or insect or jellyfish venom

A severe reaction can occur immediately or over a period of 30 minutes or more. The signs and symptoms of anaphylactic shock can include one or more of the following:

- An itching or burning sensation of the skin
- Tingling in the fingers and toes
- A rash or hives
- A feeling of tightness in the chest and throat
- Noisy breathing or wheezing
- Difficulty breathing
- Nausea and diarrhea
- Fainting
- Unconsciousness
- Dizziness
- Swelling of any or all of the following:
  - Face
  - Neck
  - Lips
  - Tongue

Use the following steps if you think someone is having a severe allergic reaction:

1. Call for help.
2. Provide the victim with prescribed medication, if available. People who know they are severely allergic often carry an epinephrine autoinjector (syringe) in case of a reaction.
3. Monitor the victim for breathing and circulation until medical help arrives.

CONCERNS FOR PREGNANT WOMEN

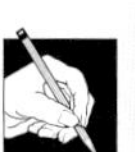

The body goes through a range of changes with pregnancy. Many of these changes are normal, but a woman should call her obstetrician if she experiences any of the following symptoms:

- Bleeding or fluid leaking from the vagina
- Vaginal itching
- Genital sores or warts
- Blurry or impaired vision
- Unusual or severe abdominal or back pain
- Frequent, severe, or continuous headaches
- Contractions
- Dizziness
- Excessive vomiting or diarrhea
- Fever over 101 degrees Fahrenheit (38 degrees Celsius)
- Pain or burning with urination
- Strong cramps
- Swelling of the face, fingers, or feet
- Persistent chills
- Inability to tolerate foods or liquids
- Muscular convulsions
- Sudden weight gain or loss of two pounds within one day
- Fainting
- Increased thirst with decreased urination

REVIEW QUESTIONS

1. Fainting is ______________________ and the victim ______________________.
2. Asthma is a ______________________ that is marked by recurring episodes of ______________________.
3. ______________________ is a major cause of COPD.
4. Give a diabetic emergency victim ______________________ ______________________. If the victim's problem is high blood sugar, giving the victim sugar will ______________________. If the problem is hypoglycemia, giving them sugar will ______________________the symptoms.
5. Seizures can range from apparent ______________________ to blackouts to sudden and ______________________.
6. Severe allergic reactions or anaphylactic shock are ______________________ and require ______ ______________________.
7. A woman should call her obstetrician if she experiences any of the following symptoms: - list 10 of 19 symptoms from the text. ______________________
____
____
____
____
____
____
____
____
____

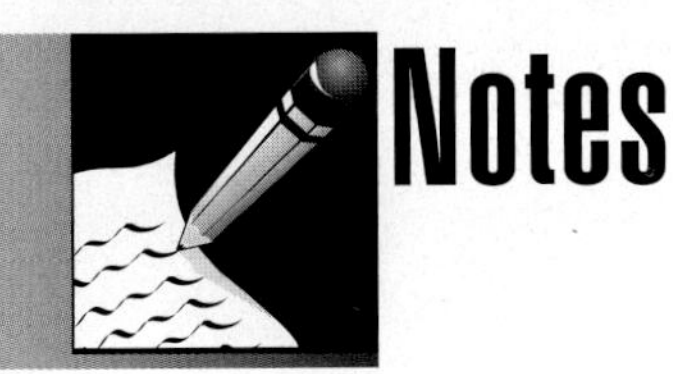

Notes

CHAPTER 15

Burns

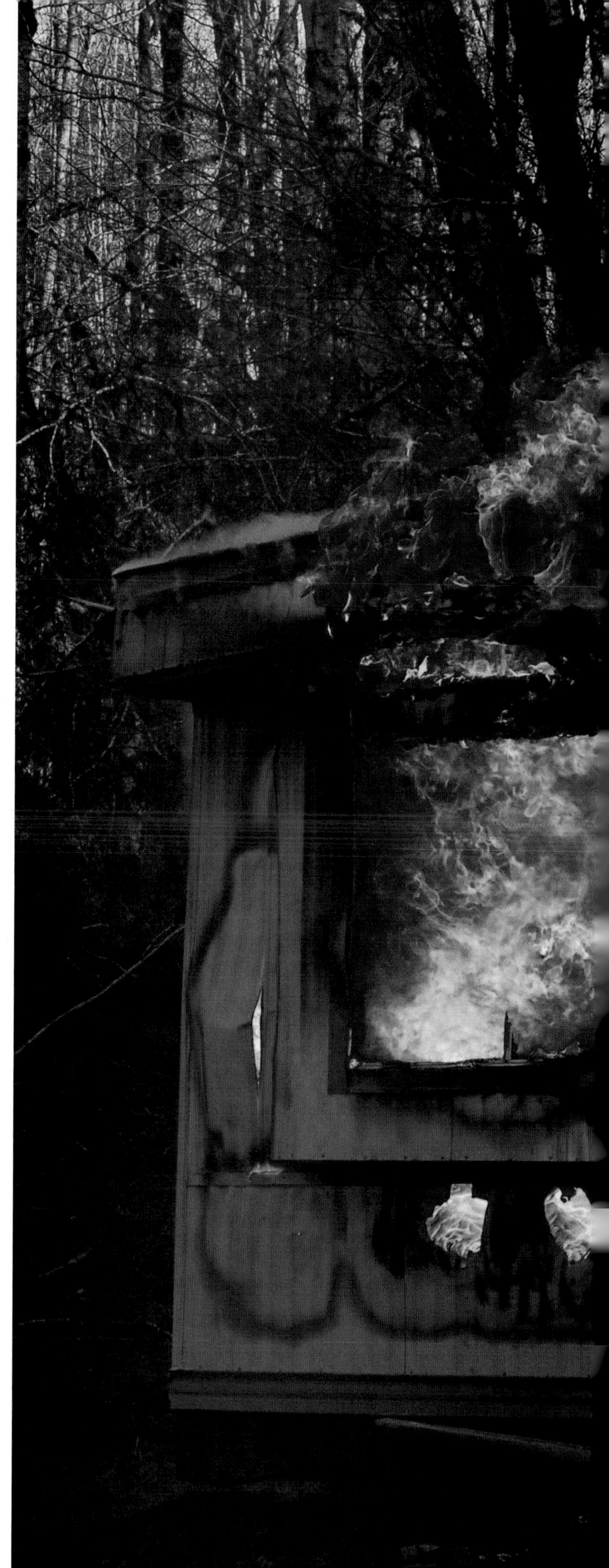

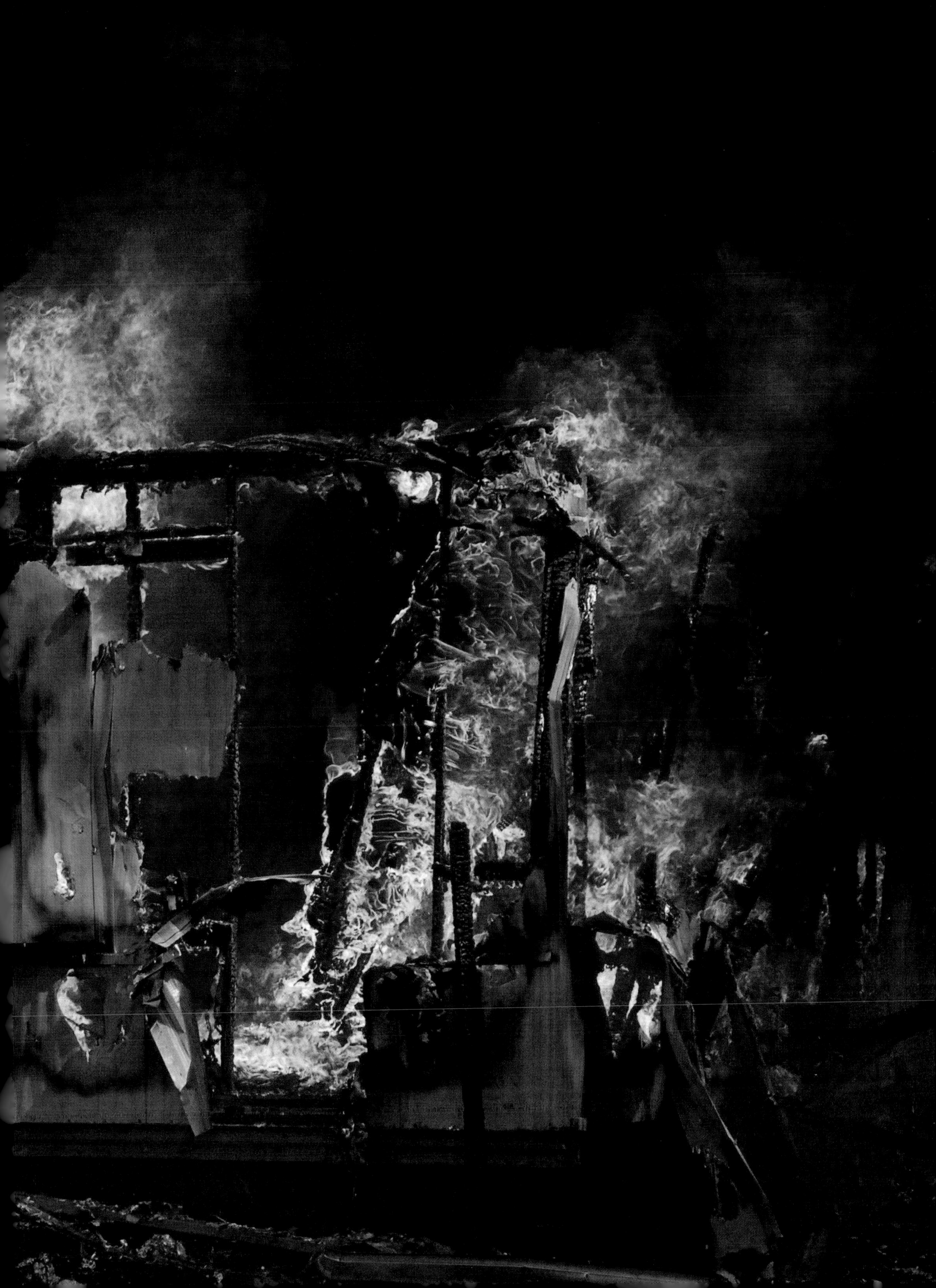

At some point, you will encounter a victim with a burn. It might be as simple as mild sunburn, or it might be much more severe such as a chemical burn that blisters the skin.

LEARNING GOALS

In this chapter you will learn about:

- Categories of burns
- Burn care by cause and severity

SEVERITY OF BURNS

Burns fall into three categories based on severity.

First Degree

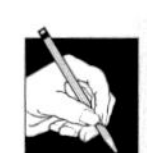

First degree or superficial burns damage only the top layer of skin. The skin is usually red and dry. The area might be swollen. These burns are painful due to damaged nerve endings. These burns usually heal in five to six days.

Second Degree

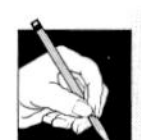

Second-degree burns or partial-thickness burns damage the top layers of skin. The skin is red and has blisters. Some of the blisters might burst, giving the skin a moist appearance. The area might be swollen. These burns are usually painful. These burns heal in three to four weeks.

Third Degree

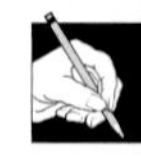

Third-degree or full-thickness burns destroy all the layers of skin and some or all of the underlying tissue (muscle, bone, fat, and nerves). These burns look brown or black and the underlying tissue might appear white. These burns can be either extremely painful or painless (if the burn has destroyed the nerve endings).

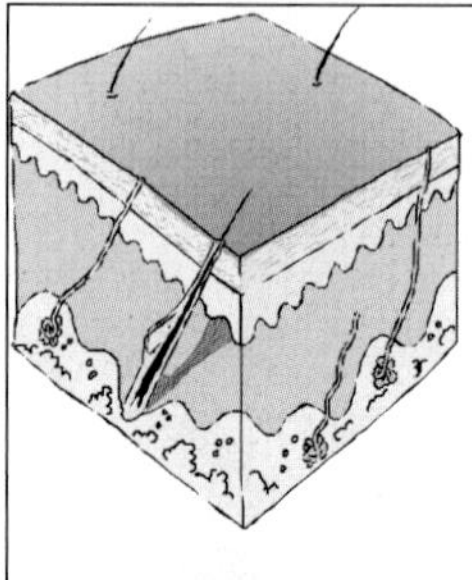

First Degree Burn
The skin is usually red and dry. The area might be swollen.

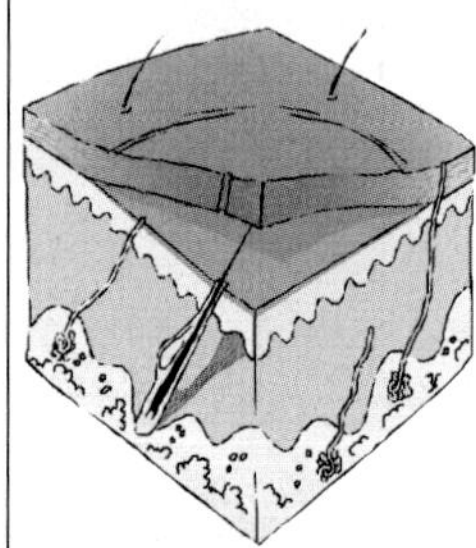

Second Degree Burn
The skin is red and has blisters. Some blisters might burst, giving the skin a moist appearance. The area might be swollen.

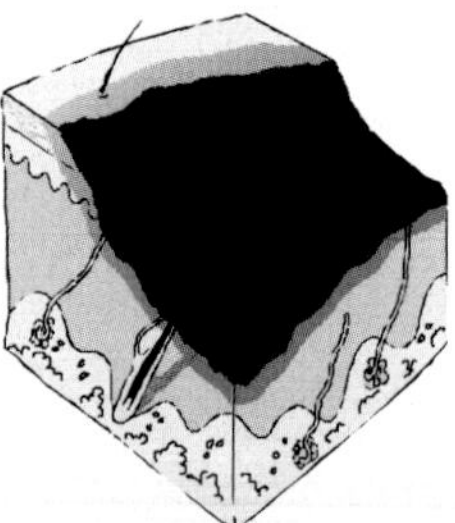

Third Degree Burn
These burns look brown or black and the underlying tissue might appear white.

Burns fall into three categories based on severity.

CAUSES OF BURNS AND THEIR FIRST AID

Burns can be caused by heat, radiation, chemicals, or electricity.

Heat Burns

Burns caused by heat are the most common. Heat burns are caused by a hot stove, flames, hot liquid, hot grease, and other heat sources. Radiation burns are most commonly caused by the sun. You cannot always tell how severe a burn is right after it has happened. Call for help if one or more of the following symptoms are present:

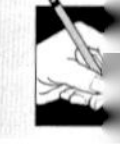

- The victim is having trouble breathing.
- The burns affect more than one area of the body.
- The burns are to the hands, feet, neck, head, or genitals (unless it is a first-degree burn).

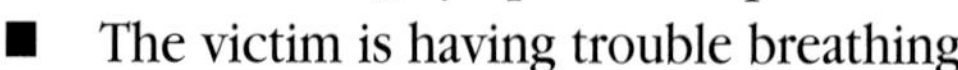

- The victim is a child or elderly person (unless it is a first-degree burn).

Use the following steps to treat first- and second-degree heat burns:

1. Cool the burned area by immersing the area in cold water or running cold water over the burn.
2. Cover the burned area with a sterile or clean, dry dressing.
3. Elevate the burned area above the level of the victim's heart.
4. Monitor for shock.

Use the following steps to treat third-degree heat burns:

1. Call for help immediately!
2. Loosely cover the burned area with a sterile or clean, dry dressing.
3. Elevate the burned area above the level of the victim's heart.
4. Treat for shock.

Remember the following recommendations when treating a burn:

- Do not apply any home remedies or ointments to a burn.
- Do not apply ice directly to the skin or burned area.
- Do not break any blisters that form.
- Do not remove any pieces of clothing or other items stuck to a burn.
- Do not apply moist dressings to a burn.
- Watch for signals and changes in breathing and consciousness.
- Keep the victim from getting chilled or overheated.
- Call for help or get the victim to medical attention if necessary.

Chemical Burns

Certain chemicals used in laboratories or other industries can cause burns. Household cleaners, paint remover, and bleach are examples of some of the chemicals you have in your house that can cause chemical burns. The stronger the chemical and the longer the chemical stays on the skin, the more severe the burn. With a chemical burn, you want to remove the burning agent quickly by flushing the area with water. You must call for help if you have a victim with a chemical burn.

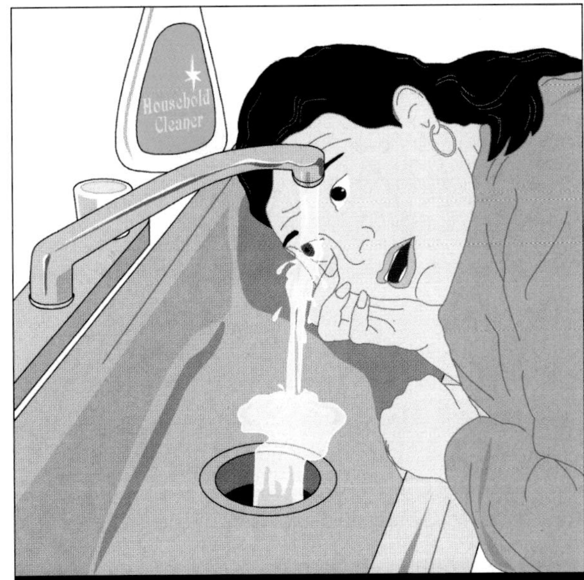

If the chemical is in or around the eye, be sure to flush the eye from the nose outward.

Use the following steps to treat chemical burns:

1. Call for help.
2. Wash the burned area with gently flowing water for at least 20 minutes. Remove any contaminated clothing or jewelry during this time.
   NOTE: If the chemical is in or around the eye, be sure to flush the eye from the nose outward so that you don't wash the chemical over the nose and into the other eye.
3. Treat for shock.

Electrical Burns

Electrical burns can be caused by electrical wires or from lightning. The severity of the burn depends on the length of time the victim was in contact with the current, and the strength and type of current. The victim will have two wounds - one where the electricity entered the body and one where the electricity exited the

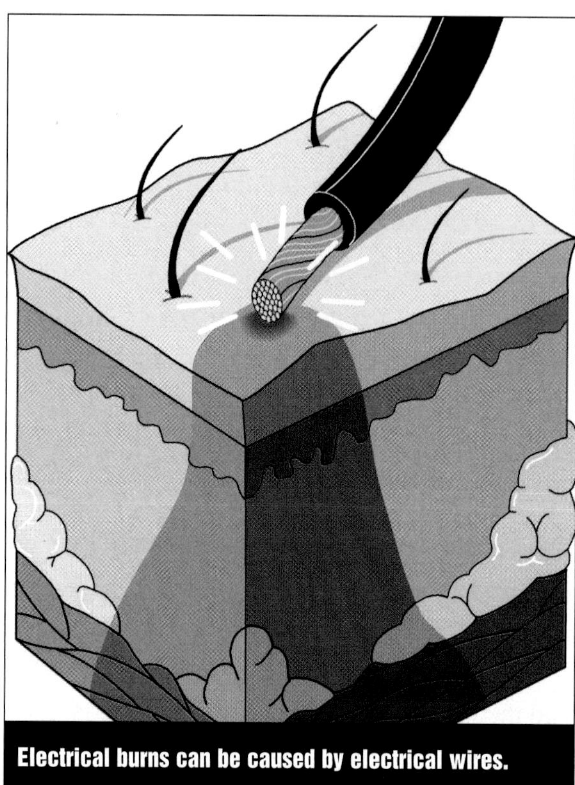

Electrical burns can be caused by electrical wires.

body. The visible wounds might be small, but there can be extensive tissue damage internally. Use the following steps to treat electrical burns:

1. Call for help!
2. Be sure the power is turned off before approaching the victim. (Check the immediate area for a main electrical breaker that can cut power to the vicinity, or use a non-conductive material, such as a wooden broom handle, to remove the electrical source from the victim.)
3. Check for airway and breathing and provide the appropriate care.
4. Do not move the victim unless absolutely necessary. There is a chance of spinal trauma from the electrical discharge.
5. Cover the burned area with a sterile or clean, dry dressing.
6. Treat for shock.

REVIEW QUESTIONS

1. First degree or superficial burns damage ________________________________.

2. Second-degree burns or partial-thickness burns damage________________________.

3. Third-degree or full-thickness burns ________________________________

____.

4. Radiation burns are most commonly caused by ____________________________.

5. ____ are examples of some of the chemicals you have in your house that can cause chemical burns.

6. When responding to a victim of an electrical burn, ______________________________ ______________________________ before approaching the victim.

Notes

CHAPTER 16

Heat and Cold Emergencies

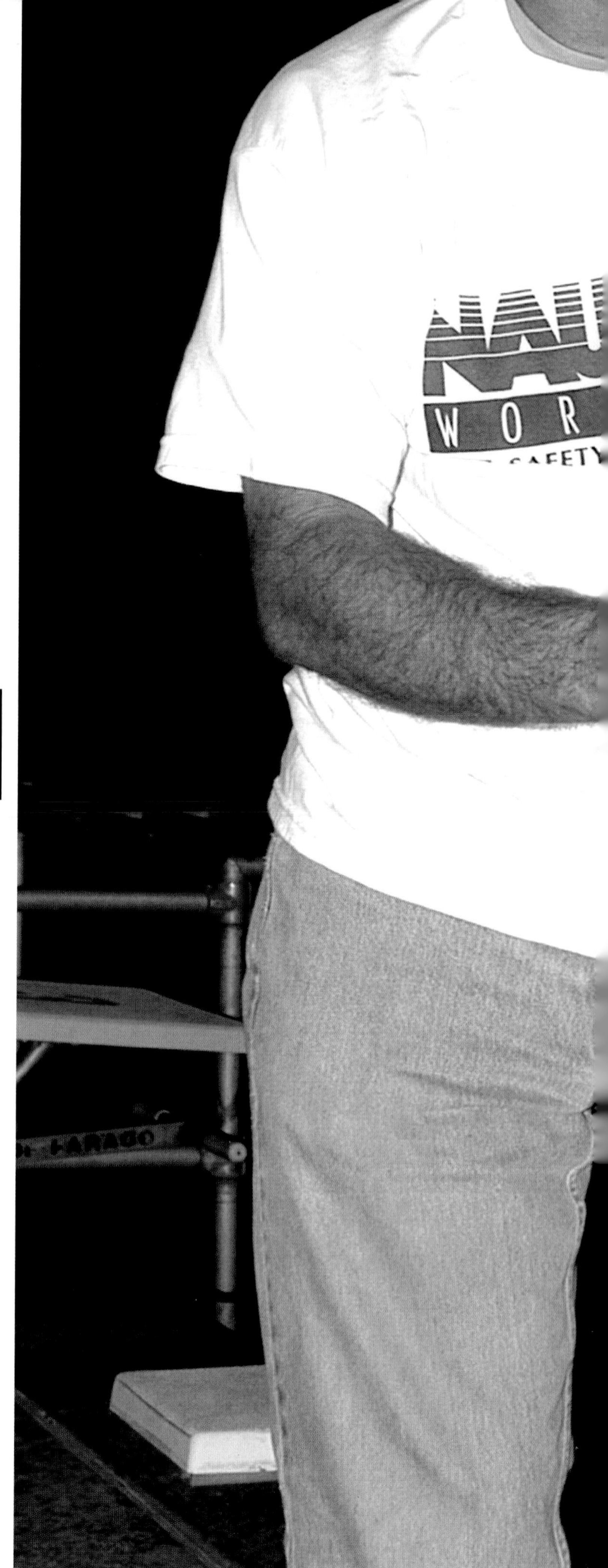

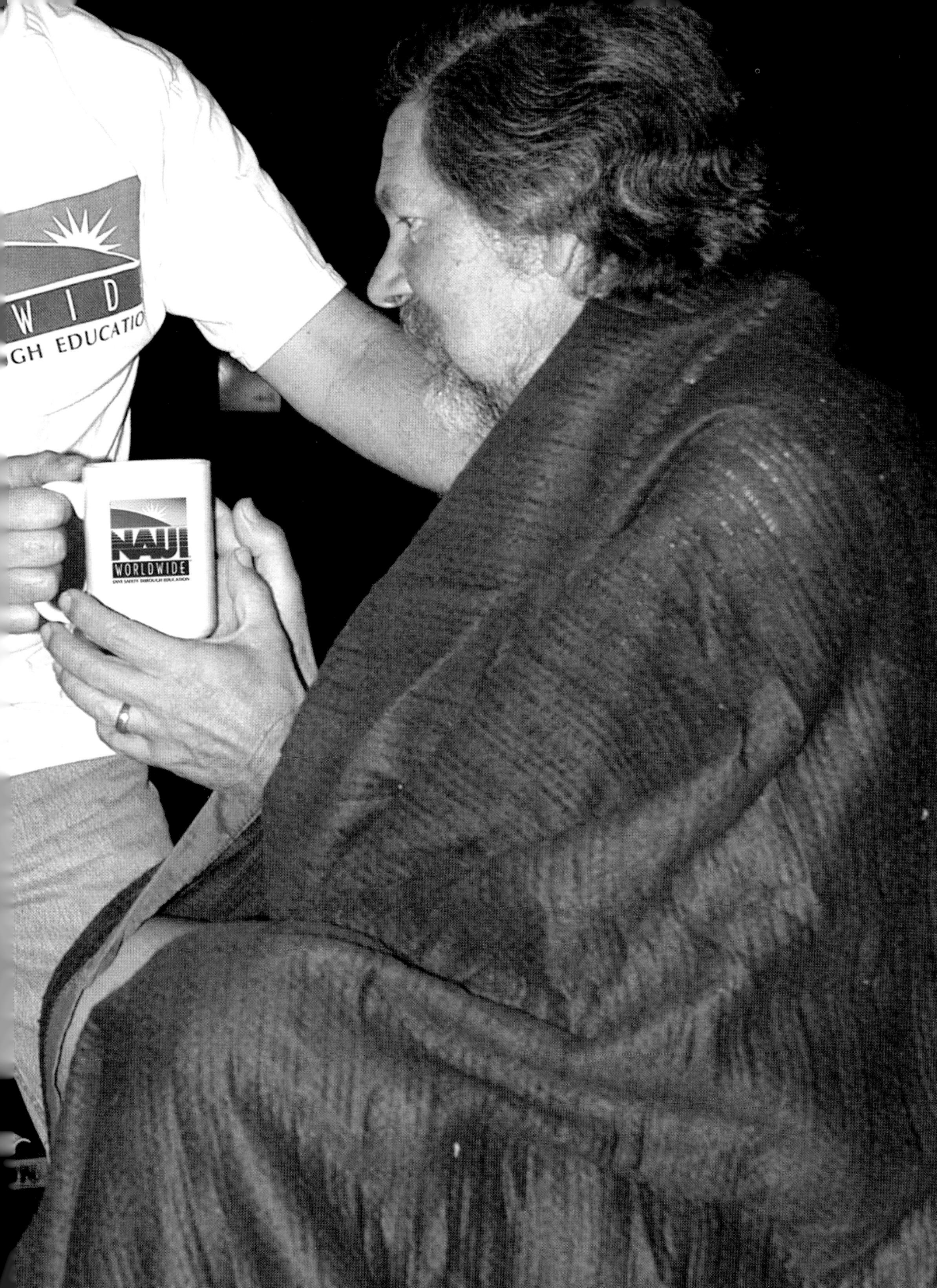
NAUI
WORLDWIDE

Exposure to extreme heat or cold without adequate insulation, adequate heat dissipation (in the heat) or adequate heat generation (in the cold) can make you ill.

LEARNING GOALS

In this chapter you will learn about:

- Hyperthermia: heat cramps, heat exhaustion, and heat stroke
- Hypothermia: chilling (mild), clinical (severe), and frostbite
- Immersion foot

HEAT AND COLD RISK

People at risk for heat- or cold-related illnesses are:

- Those who only work or exercise indoors so that they are unaccustomed to hot or cold environments and are not acclimated
- The elderly
- Young children
- Those with health problems

Once someone begins to show signs or symptoms of a heat- or cold-related illness, their condition will continue to worsen unless first aid is administered. In some instances first aid may only require that they be removed from the environment that is causing the problem.

HYPERTHERMIA

Hyperthermia means increased (hyper) temperature (thermia). Hyperthermia can cause three different injuries:

- Heat cramps
- Heat exhaustion
- Heat stroke

Heat Cramps

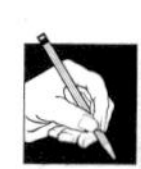

Heat cramps is an injury that affects the muscles. The signs and symptoms of heat cramps include:

- Painful muscle spasms or cramps, especially in the legs and abdomen
- Heavy sweating
- Cool, moist skin

Use the following steps to treat heat cramps:

1. Move the victim to a cool place
2. Give the victim cool water or a sports beverage to drink
3. Stretch the affected muscle back to resting length

Heat Exhaustion

Anyone working or exercising in a hot or hot and humid environment should be aware of the symptoms of heat exhaustion and how to treat them. The signs and symptoms of heat exhaustion include:

- Cold and clammy skin
- Heavy sweating
- Weakness and fatigue
- Headache
- Nausea
- Weak pulse
- Shallow breathing

Use the following steps to treat heat exhaustion:

1. Move the victim to a cool place.
2. Settle them in a comfortable position.
3. Loosen tight clothing.
4. Remove any sweat-soaked clothing with permission.
5. Apply cool, wet cloths to the neck, armpits, and groin areas.
6. Fan the victim.
7. Give the victim cool water to drink, if they are not nauseated.
8. Monitor the victim's condition.
9. Call for more advanced help if necessary.

Heat Stroke

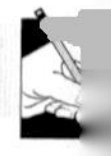

Heat stroke is a life-threatening condition. In heat stroke, the body is overwhelmed with the heat and its cooling mechanisms stop functioning.

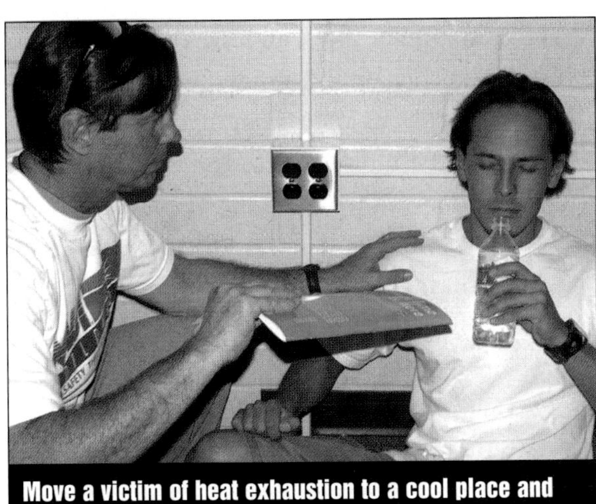

Move a victim of heat exhaustion to a cool place and give them water to drink, if they are not nauseated.

The signs and symptoms of heat stroke include:

- Red, hot, dry skin
- Confusion or changes in consciousness
- Rapid pulse
- Shallow breathing

Use the following steps to treat heat stroke:

1. Call for help immediately.
2. Move the victim to a cool place.
3. Apply cool, wet cloths to the neck, armpits, and groin areas.
4. Fan the victim.
5. Remove any excess clothing with permission.
6. Monitor the victim's condition until help arrives.

HYPOTHERMIA

- Chilling (Mild Hypothermia)
- Clinical (Severe) Hypothermia
- Frostbite

Hypothermia means decreased (hypo) temperature (thermia). The entire body cools because its ability to generate enough heat to keep warm is overcome by the cold environment. Hypothermia can be mild or severe. The sooner you recognize the signs and symptoms of hypothermia and provide care, the better the chance that the condition will not worsen.

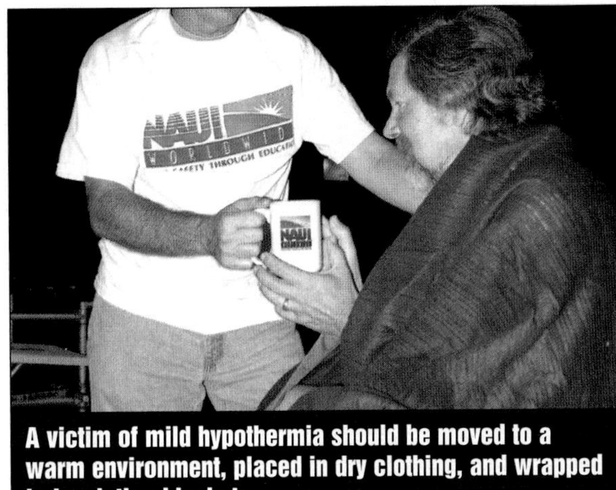

A victim of mild hypothermia should be moved to a warm environment, placed in dry clothing, and wrapped in insulating blankets.

Mild Hypothermia

Mild hypothermia can occur when someone:

- Has been in cold water
- Has stayed in wet clothing
- Has ingested substances, such as alcohol, that interfere with the body's response to cold
- Has a condition that impairs their circulation, such as cardiovascular disease or diabetes

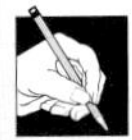

The signs and symptoms of mild hypothermia include:

- Shivering
- Numbness
- Apathy
- Stumbling or staggering

Use the following steps to care for mild hypothermia:

1. Move the victim to a warmer environment.
2. Replace wet clothing with dry clothing.
3. Wrap the victim in blankets, coats, or any available insulator.
4. Give the victim warm liquids to drink if they are conscious.

Do not try to warm the victim too quickly–for example, putting them in a hot bath. Rapid re-warming can cause heart problems or secondary cooling as blood vessels in the extremities dilate and still-cool blood is shunted to the trunk of the body.

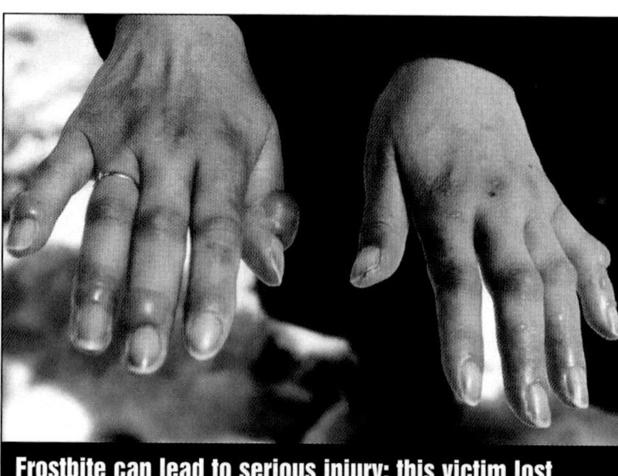
Frostbite can lead to serious injury; this victim lost portions of three fingers.

Severe Hypothermia

Severe hypothermia can occur when someone has been exposed to the cold for an extended period of time. The signs and symptoms of severe hypothermia include:

- Still and rigid muscles
- No sign of shivering
- Skin looks blue and victim does not react to pain
- Pulse and respirations are very slow or might not be able to be detected
- Pupils are dilated

Use the following steps to care for severe hypothermia:

1. Call for help immediately.
2. Keep the victim from getting any colder.
3. Do not actively re-warm the victim unless you are in a remote location and transport to a medical facility will be delayed.
4. Treat the victim as if they might break when you are moving them.
5. Monitor the victim for airway, breathing, and circulation.

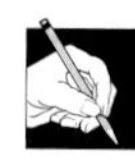

Frostbite

Frostbite is the freezing of a body area. It occurs when the area is exposed to the cold. The blood flow to the area slows down, and the body can no longer keep the area warm. Ice crystals start to form under the skin. The severity of the frostbite depends on the air temperature, the length of exposure, and the strength of the wind. The signs and symptoms of frostbite include:

- White and waxy skin appearance
- Lack of feeling in the affected area
- Skin that can feel frozen to the touch

Use the following steps to care for frostbite:

1. Move the victim to a warmer environment.
2. Unless there is a possibility that it might refreeze, rewarm the affected part by placing it in water no warmer than 105° Fahrenheit (40° Celsius).
3. Keep the area in the water until color returns and the skin feels warm.
4. Once the area thaws, cover it with a sterile dressing and place padding between fingers and toes.
5. Transport the victim to a medical facility.

IMMERSION FOOT

Immersion foot (trench foot) occurs when your feet are subjected to cold and wet conditions for long periods of time. This can happen when backpacking and camping. The signs and symptoms of immersion foot include:

- Cold and blotchy skin
- Numbness
- Tingling
- Prickling or a wooden feeling in the foot
- Bounding pulse in the foot
- Red, dry, and painful foot once it becomes warm

Use the following steps to prevent immersion foot:

1. Dry your feet and put on dry socks daily. Use a pair of socks that wick moisture away from your skin. You can additionally wear a pair of wool socks to keep your feet warm and insulated in cold weather.

2. Dry your shoes or boots aggressively when they have been immersed in water. Keep them in the sun or near a heat source.
3. Sleep without socks on to allow your feet to air out. If necessary, wrap your feet in an article of clothing for warmth.
4. Check your feet daily for signs and symptoms of immersion foot.

REVIEW QUESTIONS

1. The signs and symptoms of heat cramps include: - list 2 of 3 signs or symptoms from the text.

   ____

   ____

2. The signs and symptoms of heat exhaustion include: - list 4 of 7 signs or symptoms from the text.

   ____

   ____

   ____

   ____

3. Heat stroke is ______________________________.

4. Hypothermia means ______________________________.

5. The signs and symptoms of mild hypothermia include: - list 3 of 4 signs or symptoms from the text. ______________________________

   ____

   ____

6. Do not actively re-warm a victim of severe hypothermia unless ______________________________

   ______________________________.

7. ______________________________ occurs when your ______________________________ are subjected to cold and wet conditions for long periods of time.

CHAPTER 17

Water Hazards

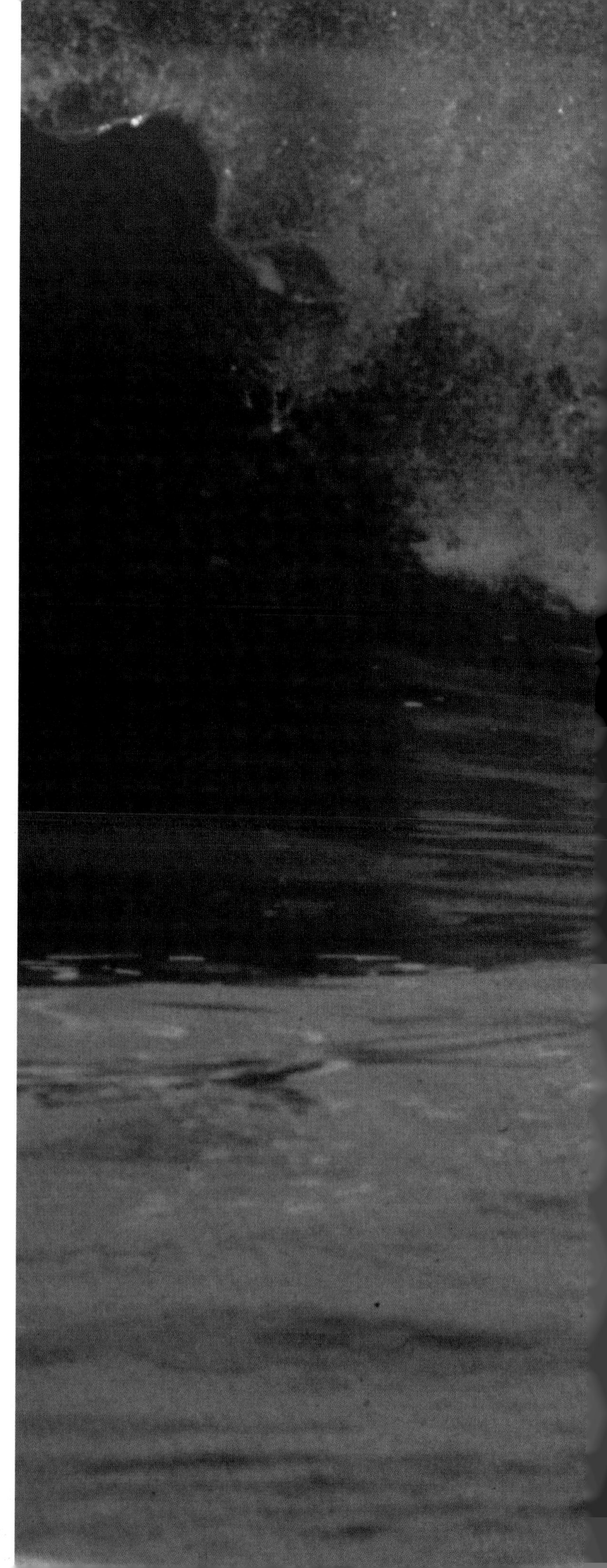

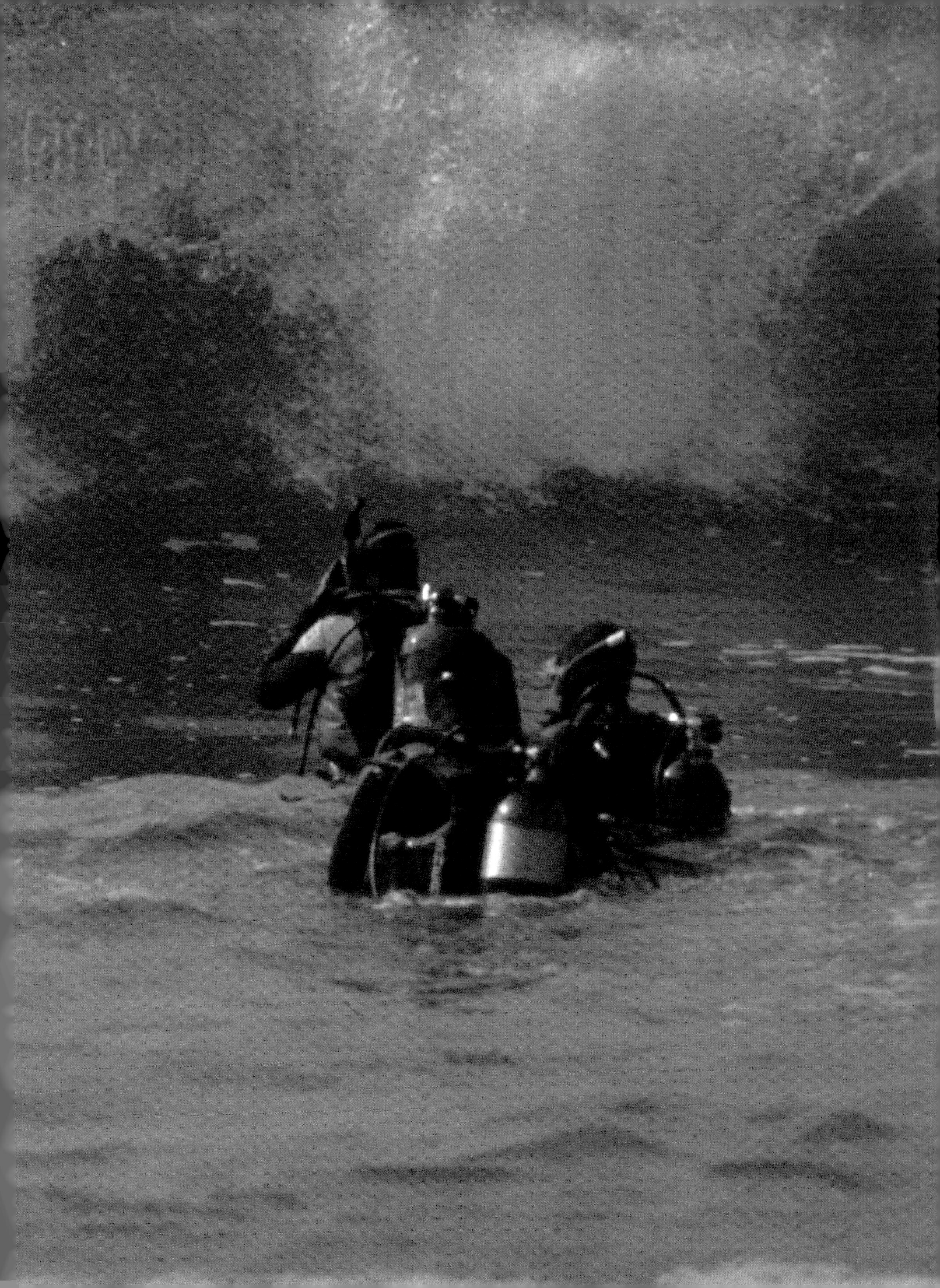

Water hazards include drowning (or near-drowning) from accidental immersion or while participating in water recreations, such as swimming or water skiing. Other water hazards include pressure related injuries while skin or scuba diving and contact with venomous or hazardous aquatic life.

LEARNING GOALS

In this chapter you will learn about:

- Drowning and near-drowning
- Cold water drowning
- Skin and scuba diving maladies
- Aquatic life injuries

DROWNING AND NEAR-DROWNING

Drowning is death caused by suffocation due to submersion or immersion in a liquid, usually water or seawater. Drowning is the second leading cause of unintended death worldwide following auto/traffic related deaths, and the leading cause of accidental death of children under five years old.

The first aid for drowning or near-drowning victims is the same until advanced medical assistance arrives. In the event that a victim is revived as a result of resuscitation, it is important that they be evaluated by emergency medical personnel or a physician because of the potential for delayed, life-threatening onset of symptoms. Some of the signs and symptoms of drowning include:

- Unconscious victim in or near a body of water
- Cessation of breathing
- Absence of a pulse
- Cyanosis (bluish lips and fingernail beds)
- Confusion
- Coughing or spitting up fluid that is pink or frothy

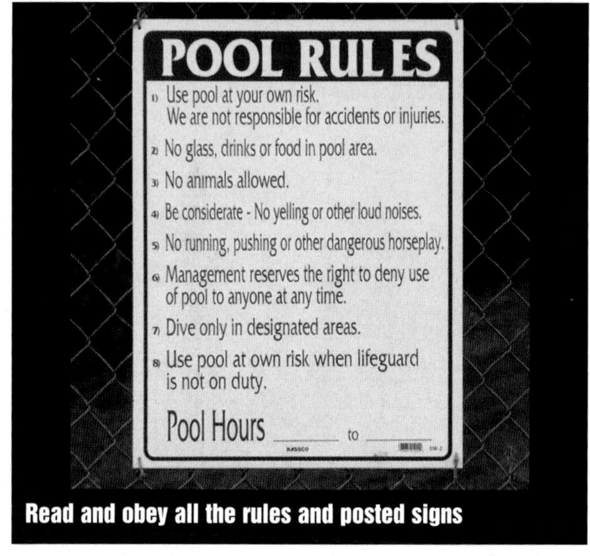

Read and obey all the rules and posted signs

- Abdominal swelling
- Vomiting

After you have evaluated the scene, use the following steps to care for a drowning victim:

1. Remove the victim from the water. (Victim transport techniques are explained elsewhere in this text.)
2. Follow the steps for rescue breathing and CPR if needed.
3. If the victim is conscious perform a secondary survey and monitor until they can be referred to emergency medical personnel or a physician for care and observation.

Use the following steps to prevent drowning:

1. Learn to swim and encourage enrolling in learn-to-swim programs by children, adolescents, and adults.
2. Never swim alone - always swim with a buddy.
3. Install child safety barriers around swimming pools, and use locking covers on hot tubs and spas.
4. Be careful of long hair getting caught in suction drains in hot tubs and spas (especially on children playing breath-hold games).
5. Provide competent supervision for all aquatic-related recreational activities.

6. Prohibit the use of alcohol at any aquatic recreational activity. (Be especially wary of consuming alcohol prior to using a hot tub or spa.)
7. In open water, always distance-swim parallel to shore and near a lifeguard. Don't overestimate your swimming ability.
8. If caught in a current swim out of the current by swimming across it and then return to shore.
9. Never dive headfirst into the water unless the area is clearly marked and designated for diving.
10. Read and obey all the rules and posted signs.
11. Children and weak swimmers should always wear an approved personal flotation device (PFD) when aboard a boat or around the water.

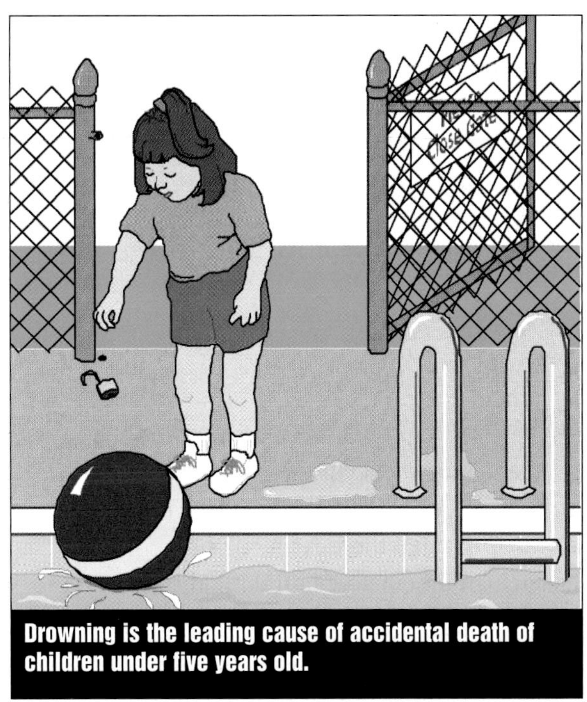

Drowning is the leading cause of accidental death of children under five years old.

COLD-WATER DROWNING

Submersion in cold water can also induce the rapid onset of hypothermia, which has been observed to extend the time after clinical death during which a victim may be successfully revived and survive to return to normal life activities. This phenomenon is affected by many factors such as age, time, temperature, intracellular pH, metabolic rate, biochemical changes, high-energy storage deposits, as well as institution of re-warming techniques. Younger victims have been revived after an hour of submersion. Although still not fully understood, in the case of cold-water drowning advanced medical care and re-warming in a clinical setting is recommended even after prolonged submersion.

SKIN AND SCUBA DIVING MALADIES

As certified divers learn in their first diving course, the pressure of the water affects the body's air spaces. The increased pressure when diving also causes in-gassing of nitrogen, which can also cause problems if divers fail to follow the basic rules of scuba diving.

BAROTRAUMAS (PRESSURE INJURIES)

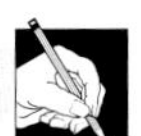

A barotrauma is any injury due to pressure. Any closed air space in your body or closed air space created by your equipment (mask or dry suit) will subject you to injury if the pressure inside the air space is too much different from the surrounding or ambient pressure and you cannot equalize the pressure. The major categories of barotraumas are:

- Squeezes
- Reverse blocks
- Eardrum rupture
- Round window rupture
- Pulmonary barotrauma

SQUEEZES

Squeezes happen during descent, that is, when external pressure increases. They occur when the pressure outside an air space is greater than the pressure inside the air space and the pressure compresses or tries to compress the air space. Squeezes can occur in the following bodily or equipment air spaces when diving:

- Ears
- Sinuses
- Mask
- Tooth
- Dry suit

Ears

Ear squeezes occur when a diver does not equalize their ears on descent. They can also occur when there is any blockage of the Eustachian tube between the middle ear and the throat that does not allow the diver to clear their ears. If a diver ignores an ear squeeze and continues to descend, they can rupture an eardrum. The signs and symptoms of an ear squeeze include:

- Discomfort in the ear, ranging up to extreme pain
- Dullness of sounds, such as exhalation bubbles underwater
- A feeling of fullness in the ear upon surfacing

You can easily prevent an ear squeeze by equalizing your ears early and often on a controlled descent. This is something diving students learn and practice in their initial training. To review:

- Equalizing one's ears is best done immediately upon submerging and often throughout a descent so that pressure never builds up too much.
- Use a gentle exhalation pressure with a closed mouth and pinched nose. Some also find it easy to use the tongue as a piston to compress the air in the back of the mouth and gently force it into the Eustachian tubes to offset the increasing external pressure as you descend.
- Using a descent or anchor line also aids in controlling the rate of descent and allows halting it altogether to allow for easy equalization.

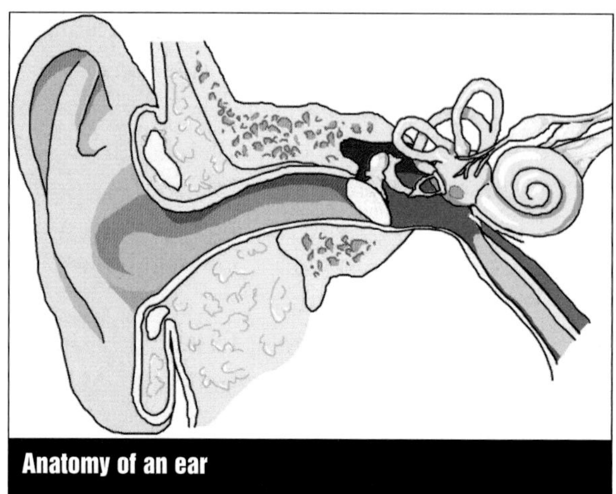

Anatomy of an ear

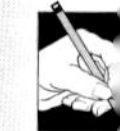

However, you should not force the equalization of your ears if equalizing is difficult. You should not dive when you are suffering from a cold or allergies. When you have a cold or allergies, you can have mucus in your Eustachian tubes or the tissue in the tubes could be swollen. When you try to equalize, you can force mucus as well as air into your middle ear. This can cause a middle ear infection.

If you do feel an ear squeeze while diving, use the following steps to clear the squeeze:

1. Ascend a short distance, even just a foot or two (half a meter).
2. Attempt to gently equalize your ears. If you are successful, go to step 3. If you are not successful, repeat step 1.
3. Descend slightly and equalize again. If your ears equalize, continue your descent, equalizing gently and frequently as your descend.

If you cannot equalize, you must end your dive and return to the surface. If you have a feeling of fullness in one or both ears, you may have fluid in your middle ear as a result of your body's attempts to reduce the size of the trapped air space. You should seek medical attention.

Sinuses

Sinuses are air-filled cavities in your head that open into your nasal passages. In healthy sinuses, air can move freely in and out through the openings. Sinus squeezes occur when mucus has blocked the openings, and air is trapped in the sinus cavities. The mucus plug is usually a result of a cold, infection, or allergies. The signs and symptoms of a sinus squeeze include:

- Sharp, stabbing pain above or under the eyes
- Pain in the upper teeth around the incisors, similar to a toothache
- Blood in the mask; this is usually not noticed until after surfacing

Preventing sinus squeezes is simple. Do not dive when you have nasal congestion from a cold, infection, or allergies. Use the following steps if you feel a sinus squeeze:

1. Ascend and end your dive.
2. Inhale warm, steamy air, or place a warm, wet facecloth over your forehead, eyes, and cheekbones to help clear the blockage.
3. If the pain is not resolved, seek medical attention.

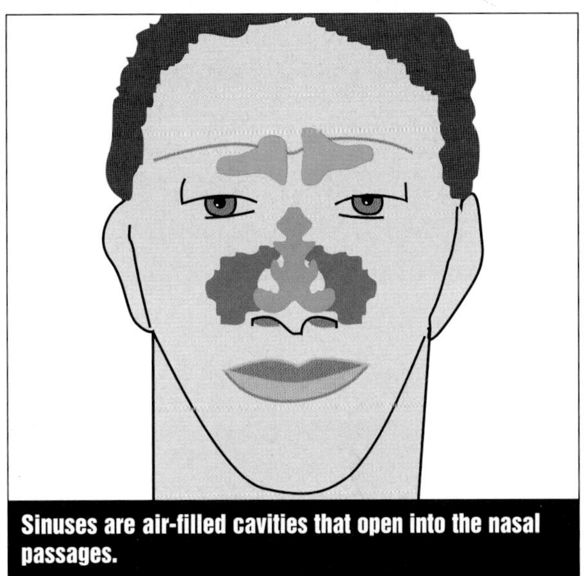

Sinuses are air-filled cavities that open into the nasal passages.

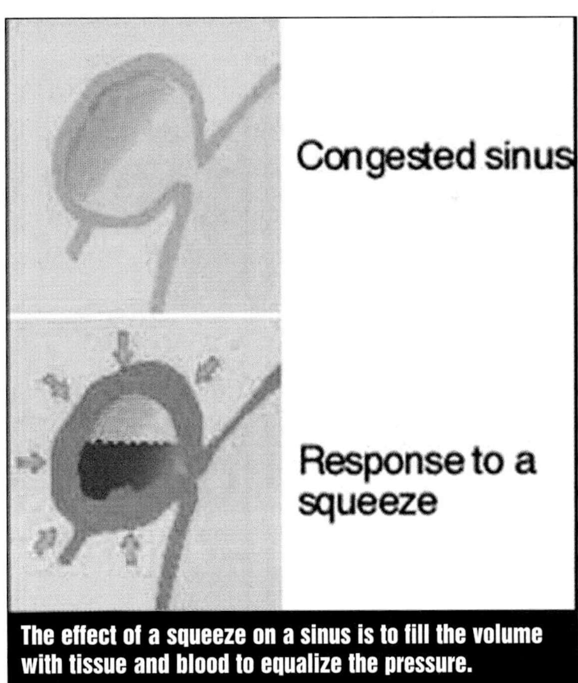

The effect of a squeeze on a sinus is to fill the volume with tissue and blood to equalize the pressure.

Mask

Your mask creates an air space between your face and the mask itself. You must remember to equalize this air space as you descend by periodically exhaling a small amount of air through your nose. If you do not equalize the air space, the mask will begin to feel like a suction cup pulling your eyes, nose, and surrounding skin into the mask. Simply breathe out through your nose occasionally as you descend to equalize the pressure between your face and the mask.

If you do not equalize the air space between the mask and your face, a severe mask squeeze can cause:

- Bloodshot eyes from rupturing the blood vessels of the whites of your eyes
- Bruising of the face area enclosed by the mask

Use the following steps if you experience a mask squeeze:

1. Place an ice pack on the area to help relieve the pain and swelling.
2. Seek medical attention if the bruising and swelling are severe.

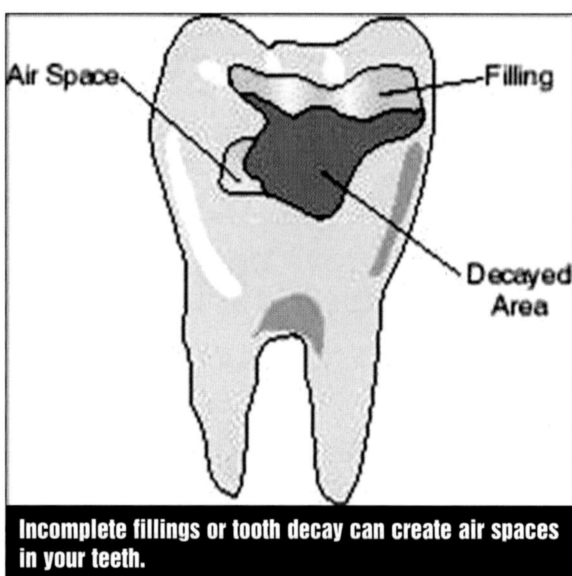

Incomplete fillings or tooth decay can create air spaces in your teeth.

Tooth

Incomplete fillings or tooth decay can create air spaces in your teeth. You will feel pain in the tooth if you have a tooth squeeze. Ignoring the squeeze could result in bleeding or a broken tooth. Use the following steps if you feel a tooth squeeze:

1. End your dive.
2. Go to a dentist, preferably one who understands diving, to have your tooth repaired.

Dry Suit

A dry suit creates an air space around your body. The air space warms up to your body temperature, and along with the dry suit undergarment you wear, keeps you warm. If you do not have any air in the air space, you feel as if you are encased in a vacuum bag. Increasing water pressure can compress folds in the suit against your skin and cause painful pinches. Dry suits are equipped with a low-pressure inflator valve so you can add air to the dry suit to equalize the pressure. If you feel pinching, you can also shift the air within the suit to relieve the pinch.

REVERSE BLOCKS

Reverse blocks occur during ascent if the pressure inside an air space becomes greater than the pressure outside the air space. Reverse blocks can occur in the following air spaces when diving:

- Ears
- Sinuses

Ears

Reverse blocks in the ear occur when there is a blockage of the Eustachian tube between the middle ear and the throat. The blockage is usually a result of diving with congestion from a cold or allergies. As you ascend, the air in the middle ear expands, but it cannot escape because of the blockage. This causes first a sensation of fullness and then a sharp pain in your ear. If you ignore a reverse block, you can cause your eardrum to rupture or damage the membranes separating the middle and inner ear. If you experience some dizziness after ascent, this can be due to unequal clearing of your ears (alternobaric vertigo). Use the following steps if you experience a reverse block in your ear during an ascent from a dive:

1. Descend a short distance until comfort is restored.
2. Gently equalize your ears.
3. Ascend slowly, allowing your ears to equalize. If your ears will not equalize, ascend as slowly as possible.
4. If necessary, seek medical treatment from a specialist who is familiar with or has experience in diving medicine.

Sinuses

Reverse blocks in the sinuses occur when mucus traps expanding air in the sinuses. The blockage is often a result of taking decongestants to clear congestion from a cold or allergies, and the decongestant wears off during the dive. As you ascend, the air in the sinus expands, but cannot escape because of the blockage. This causes a sharp pain that is usually felt behind the eyes. Use the following steps if you experience a reverse block in your sinuses during an ascent from a dive:

1. Descend a short distance until the pain subsides.
2. Ascend slowly in small increments, allowing your sinuses to equalize. If your sinuses will not equalize, ascend as slowly as possible.
3. If necessary, seek medical treatment from a specialist who is familiar with or has experience in diving medicine.

EARDRUM RUPTURE

Ignoring an ear squeeze or block can "break" an eardrum when the pressure differential becomes too great. Usually, water will enter the middle ear through the tear. The pain of the block will suddenly stop, but the cool water on the ruptured side will cause a temperature difference between the middle and inner ears and immediate vertigo (extreme dizziness) will result. If this happens, hold onto any stable object - even your dive partner - until the vertigo passes. Then exit the water and seek medical attention.

ROUND WINDOW RUPTURE

If a diver attempts to clear their ears too forcefully, the back-pressure can cause the flexible round window between the middle ear and the inner ear to tear, and fluid will begin to leak from the inner ear. The nerve endings for hearing as well as the semicircular canals, which provide our sense of balance, are located in our inner ears. The signs and symptoms of round window rupture include:

- Tinnitus (ringing in the ear)
- Vertigo
- Loss of hearing

Round window rupture is a serious condition that normally requires surgical repair. Seek medical attention.

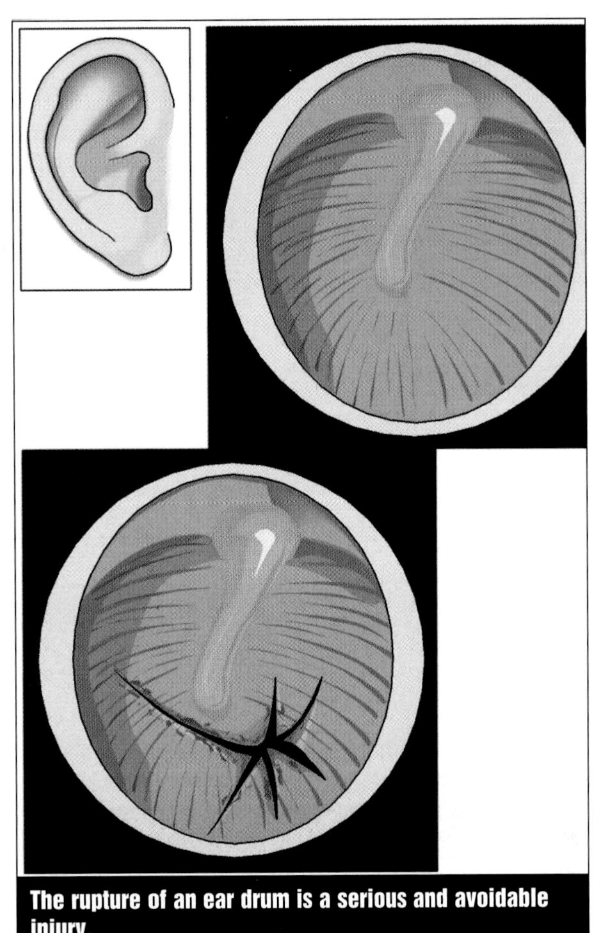

The rupture of an ear drum is a serious and avoidable injury.

PULMONARY BAROTRAUMA

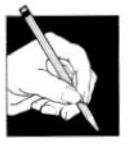

Pulmonary barotraumas (lung overexpansion injuries) occur when air expands in the lungs, and it is unable to vent through the existing lung passages. The expanding air will make its own holes through which to vent. The reason air cannot vent is usually because the diver holds their breath on ascent. Or, a diver's lungs might be damaged due to deformities, ailments, or smoking tobacco. Theoretically, pulmonary barotraumas can occur in as little as four feet of water. The prevention for pulmonary barotraumas is simple - always breathe, never hold your breath when on scuba. The types of pulmonary barotraumas are:

- Arterial gas embolism
- Pneumothorax

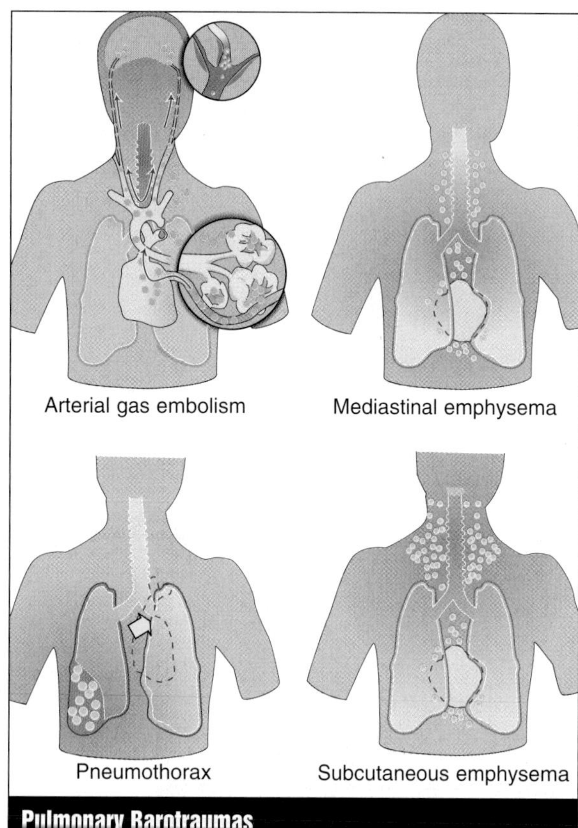

Pulmonary Barotraumas

- Mediastinal emphysema
- Subcutaneous emphysema

Arterial Gas Embolism

An arterial gas embolism (AGE) or air embolism occurs when the air escapes from the lungs into the blood stream through the pulmonary capillaries and veins. The bubbles travel in the blood through the heart to the body until they get stuck in a small artery, which blocks the blood and oxygen supply to that part of the body. An air embolism is the most serious of the lung overexpansion injuries and can cause permanent injury or death if not treated immediately.

The signs and symptoms of an air embolism normally occur within seconds to a few minutes of surfacing from a dive. The signs and symptoms of an air embolism are dependent on where the blockage occurs:

- A blockage in the brain causes symptoms of a stroke.
- A blockage in the arteries leading to the heart causes symptoms of a heart attack.

Unconsciousness without warning is the most common sign of an arterial gas embolism. Use the following steps if you think someone might have an arterial gas embolism:

1. Call for help.
2. Administer oxygen if it is available and you are trained to do so.
3. Monitor breathing and circulation.
4. Call Divers Alert Network (DAN). They will begin the communication process between you, the nearest medical facility, the nearest recompression chamber, the recompression chamber personnel, and any necessary evacuation personnel.
5. Transport the victim to the nearest medical facility with subsequent transport to a hyperbaric chamber.

Pneumothorax

A pneumothorax or collapsed lung occurs when the air escapes from the lungs into the pleural space between the lungs and the chest wall. The pressure of the air in this space, which is normally airless, causes the lung to partially or totally collapse. The signs and symptoms of a pneumothorax include:

- Chest pain
- Breathing difficulty
- Reduced chest movement on the injured side
- Leaning to the injured side

Use the following steps if you think someone might have a pneumothorax:

1. Call for help.
2. Place the victim on their side with the injured side down. This will enable more complete expansion of the uninjured lung.
3. Administer oxygen if it is available and you are trained to do so.

4. Monitor breathing and circulation.
5. Transport to a medical facility.

Mediastinal Emphysema

A mediastinal emphysema occurs when the air escapes from the lungs into the space between the lungs and the sternum (breastbone). The signs and symptoms of a mediastinal emphysema include:

- Pain under the sternum
- Difficulty breathing
- Swelling
- Collapse due to direct pressure on the heart and great vessels

Use the following steps if you think someone might have a mediastinal emphysema:

1. Call for help.
2. Administer oxygen if it is available and you are trained to do so.
3. Monitor breathing and circulation.
4. Transport to a medical facility.

Subcutaneous Emphysema

A subcutaneous emphysema occurs when the air escapes from the lungs to under the skin in the neck. This is the least serious type of lung overexpansion injury. The signs and symptoms of a subcutaneous emphysema include:

- Voice changes
- Difficulty swallowing
- Crackling under the skin of the neck

Use the following steps if you think someone might have a subcutaneous emphysema:

1. Call for help.
2. Administer oxygen if it is available and trained to do so.
3. Monitor breathing and circulation.
4. Transport to a medical facility.

DECOMPRESSION SICKNESS

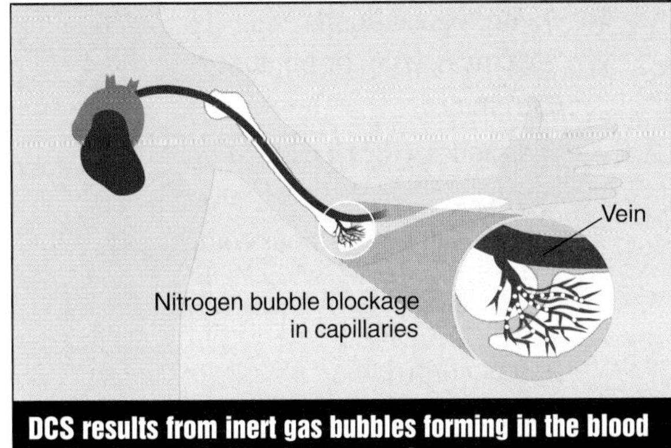

DCS results from inert gas bubbles forming in the blood and/or tissues during decompression.

As you learned in your first scuba course, decompression sickness can occur if you stay down too long and then ascend too quickly. Decompression sickness is caused by inert gas (nitrogen) that has been absorbed into your tissues during a dive coming out of solution during and after ascent and forming bubbles in your tissues.

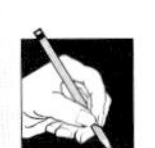

You can never eliminate the risk of decompression sickness, but you can lower that risk significantly by remembering the following:

- Do not exceed the dive time limits of your dive tables or dive computer.
- Ascend slowly - no faster than 30 feet (9 meters) per minute.
- Drink plenty of fluids and stay well hydrated.
- Make a precautionary safety stop at the end of every dive.
- Follow the recommendation of at least a one-hour surface interval between dives.

The location of the bubbles determines the signs and symptoms you have:

- Skin bends
  - Itchy skin
  - A marbled rash, commonly on the torso. This can also be a warning sign of the pending onset of serious decompression sickness.
- Limb bends
  - Joint pain. The pain can range from mild to severe.
  - Limbs and joints look normal with no swelling.

- Neurological bends
  - Weakness, pain, or numbness in the extremities
  - Pins and needles feeling in the fingers or toes
  - Extreme fatigue without comparable exertion
  - Difficult urination or loss of bladder and bowel control
  - Paralysis
  - Headache
  - Visual changes
  - Changes in mental and emotional functioning
  - Changes in personality
  - Difficulty concentrating
- Inner ear bends
  - Vertigo
  - Unsteady movement or staggering
  - Hearing loss
  - Ringing in the ears
  - Nausea
- Cardiopulmonary bends
  - The "chokes" occurs when nitrogen bubbles form in the veins of the lungs. This results in shortness of breath, chest pain, and uncontrollable coughing. This is a severe form of decompression sickness.

Use the following steps if you think someone might have decompression sickness:

1. Perform a field neurological examination. See the Section 2, Chapter 4: "Emergency Response and Victim Assessment" for the steps to performing a field neurological examination.
2. Administer oxygen if it is available and you are trained to do so.
3. Call Divers Alert Network (DAN). They will begin the communication process between you, the nearest medical facility, the nearest recompression chamber, the recompression chamber personnel, and any necessary evacuation personnel.

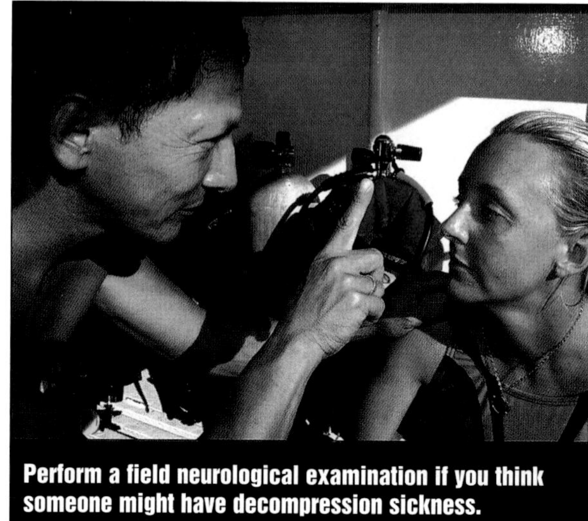

Perform a field neurological examination if you think someone might have decompression sickness.

4. Transport the victim to the nearest medical facility with subsequent transport to a hyperbaric chamber.

INDIRECT EFFECTS OF PRESSURE

You actually feel some diving maladies underwater while you are on your dive. Some of the symptoms of these maladies may still be felt after you surface. These maladies include:

- Nitrogen narcosis
- Oxygen toxicity
- Carbon dioxide toxicity

Nitrogen Narcosis

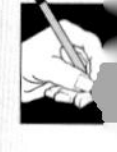

Nitrogen narcosis is a general, stuporous condition caused by breathing nitrogen gas under pressure. Nitrogen narcosis is sometimes compared to alcohol intoxication because it can present similar signs and symptoms and because of the likelihood of injury while under the influence. It usually occurs at depths greater than about 80 feet (24 meters). Symptoms increase with increasing depth. The signs and symptoms of nitrogen narcosis include:

- A reduction of mental ability
- A reduction in motor ability
- Impaired judgment and orientation

The best way to avoid nitrogen narcosis is to stay shallower than 80 feet (24 meters) when you dive. You should also be well hydrated, well rested, and avoid diving under the influence of any drugs that cause drowsiness or decrease alertness. Use the following steps if you suspect your buddy has nitrogen narcosis:

1. Have your buddy ascend a few feet.
2. Signal your buddy to see if they are okay.
3. Ascend another few feet if your buddy does not respond appropriately.

Oxygen Toxicity (Central Nervous System)

Oxygen toxicity occurs when you are exposed to elevated oxygen partial pressure. This situation usually occurs when you are breathing oxygen enriched air and go deeper than the maximum operating depth of the gas mixture. Tolerance varies, but the commonly accepted limit is 1.4 atmospheres of oxygen partial pressure. The signs and symptoms of oxygen toxicity include:

- Convulsions (these can occur without warning and cause drowning)
- Visual disturbances
- Ears ringing
- Nausea
- Twitching of the face, lips, or hands
- Irritability
- Anxiety
- Confusion
- Dizziness
- Loss of coordination
- Fatigue
- Breathing difficulty

To prevent CNS oxygen toxicity, be properly trained and certified to use oxygen enriched gas mixtures (nitrox). Analyze your gas mixture with an oxygen analyzer, do not exceed the maximum operating depth for the gas mixture you are using, and be even more conservative with increasing exertion levels.

If you suspect that you or your buddy are suffering from oxygen toxicity, end your dive and ascend to the surface.

Carbon Dioxide Toxicity

In normal breathing, there is a naturally occurring pause between the exhalation and the inhalation. A pause between the inhalation and the exhalation is a naturally occurring response to breathing underwater. Carbon dioxide build-up occurs when a diver skip breathes (pausing for an extended period after inhaling and before exhaling) or breathes too slowly. Some divers do this trying to conserve air, or have been taught this as a calming technique. Photographers may skip breathe to avoid bubbles appearing in their pictures. It is not a good technique to use while scuba diving. Carbon dioxide build-up can also occur due to breathing too rapidly and shallowly due to stress or heavy exercise. These abnormal breathing patterns can cause the carbon dioxide level in the body to increase with possible toxic effects. When the ability to detect high levels becomes blunted and the body tolerates rising levels without starting homeostatic changes to reduce it, then it builds to unhealthy levels. The signs and symptoms of carbon dioxide toxicity include:

- Respiratory discomfort
- Dizziness
- Faulty mental processes
- Stupor
- Unconsciousness without warning
- Headache upon surfacing

To prevent carbon dioxide toxicity, avoid skip breathing, shallow breathing, or excessively slow or rapid breathing when diving. Use the following steps if you suspect you or your buddy is suffering carbon dioxide toxicity:

1. End your dive and ascend to the surface.
2. Rest and breathe fresh air.
3. Call for help if their symptoms (except the headache) do not go away after breathing fresh air.

OUTER EAR INFECTIONS

When residual water from being submerged creates a hospitable environment in your outer ear canal for bacteria or fungus to grow, outer ear infections (otitis externa) or swimmer's ear can occur. The signs and symptoms of an outer ear infection include:

- Itching in your ear canal
- Pain in your ear canal and under your ear, increasing if you pull on the earlobe
- A feeling of fullness in the ear
- Hearing impairment
- Drainage from your ear

To prevent an outer ear infection, keep the ear canal's natural defenses against infection working well. Leave earwax in the canal. If earwax appears to affect your hearing or hurt your ear, see your physician. Keep your ears as dry as possible. After diving, dry your ears well. Turn your head to each side and pull the earlobe in different directions to help water run out. There are also over the counter ear drop products for drying the ear after swimming that use an alcohol and 3% boric acid solution that can help prevent swimmer's ear and infections. Use the following steps if you suspect you have an outer ear infection:

1. See your physician.
2. Follow the instructions for the medication your physician prescribes. Be sure to use the medication for the length of time your physician prescribes. The infection can re-occur if you stop using the medication too soon.

SEASICKNESS

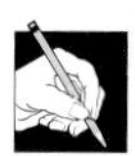

Motion, and your reaction to it, is the reason for seasickness. The amount of motion needed to trigger seasickness varies from person to person. No one is immune to seasickness, but some people have a greater resistance to it. The signs and symptoms of seasickness include:

- Unease and edginess for no apparent reason
- Pale, clammy skin
- Headache
- Weakness
- Cold sweats
- Nausea
- Vomiting

Preventing seasickness is better than trying to treat it after it occurs. Use any or all of the following suggestions to help prevent seasickness from occurring:

- Get adequate rest before your trip.
- Eat lightly and eat easily digestible foods. Greasy or salty foods are not always the best choice before a trip.
- Avoid engine exhaust fumes.
- Avoid watching or smelling others who might be sick.
- Stay in the center of the boat where the motion is the least but where you still have a good supply of fresh air.
- Avoid going below deck or into small, enclosed spaces, such as a marine toilet, unless absolutely necessary.
- Use over-the-counter remedies for seasickness, including acupressure bands or medications. If you do take a medication, start taking it the day before your trip to get it into your system.
- Take ginger (in pill form or in tea, or even fresh if you like the flavor) or eat soda crackers to help settle your stomach.

Use the following steps if you get seasick:

1. If possible, get off the boat and onto land.
2. Remain on deck and settle yourself into a spot with fresh air and as little movement as possible. Try not to fight the movement of the boat.
3. Maintain visual contact with the horizon.
4. Stay warm and hydrated.
5. Lie down and fall asleep, if possible.

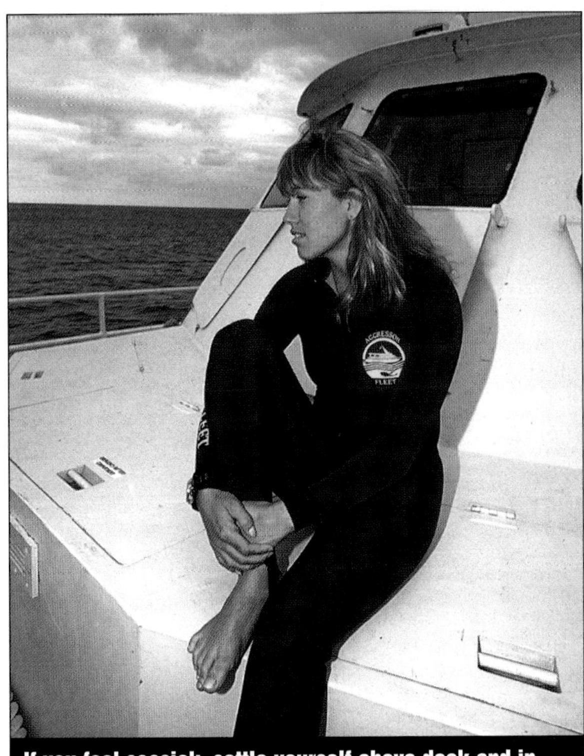

If you feel seasick, settle yourself above deck and in the center of the boat.

AQUATIC LIFE INJURIES

If you are careful and conscientious when you dive, your chance of receiving an aquatic life injury is very small. Having a "look, but don't touch" attitude towards exploring the aquatic environment will go a long way to keep you safe underwater. In general, animals attack only when they feel threatened or their territory has been invaded. If you constantly remember that you are a guest in the aquatic environment and act accordingly, you should not be the recipient of an aquatic life injury.

GENERAL CARE

The first step to care for an aquatic life injury (other than stings) is to clean the wound. Wounds in the aquatic environment are contaminated with seawater, sand, slime from aquatic animals, germs from your own skin, and other organic matter.

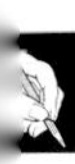

Clean the wound by irrigating it with the cleanest disinfected fresh water available. If sterile water or saline is available, that's even better to use. The force of the flow of water needs to be strong enough to dislodge any debris or bacteria but not so strong that it damages the tissue. Once the wound has been flushed, then proceed to treat it by one of the following methods:

- Heat
- Vinegar or other neutralizer
- Immobilization

The method you choose depends on the type of injury you encounter. Under each specific type of aquatic injury, you will find the preferred method of treating the injury.

Treating by Heat

Aquatic injuries where a toxin has been injected into the body by fish spines, urchins, etc. are usually treated by heat. Many toxins are heat labile, meaning the toxin is broken down in the presence of heat. Use the following steps if treating an injury with heat:

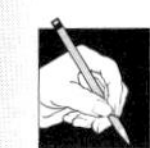

1. Immerse the wounded area in hot, but not scalding water (110° - 113° F or 43° - 45° C).
2. Keep the wounded area in the hot water for 30 to 90 minutes. Be sure the water stays as hot as the victim can tolerate it.
3. Repeat step 2 until the pain diminishes
4. For retained spines, use vinegar soaks.
5. Transport the victim to medical attention as the wound may need exploration.

Treating by White Vinegar

Aquatic injuries caused by stinging cells (nematocysts) of jellyfish, fire coral, and so on are treated with vinegar (a mild acid) to neutralize the toxin. Use the following steps if treating an injury with white vinegar:

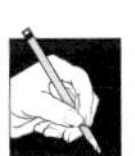

1. Rinse the area with seawater to dislodge as many nematocysts as possible.
2. Apply white vinegar to the area. Using a spray

bottle filled with vinegar wets the area without wasting the vinegar. If white vinegar is not available, use one of the following remedies:
- A paste of baking soda
- Ice packs initially then hot water

3. Scrape the stinging cells off with the edge of a credit card or dive table.
4. Reapply more vinegar to the area for 15 minutes.
5. Wash the area with soap and water.
6. Apply a thin layer of hydrocortisone cream to the area.
7. Monitor the victim for signs of an allergic reaction.
8. Transport the victim to medical attention, if necessary.

Treating by Pressure Immobilization

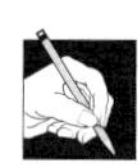

Bites from a blue-ringed octopus or a sea snake, or a puncture from a cone shell are treated with the pressure immobilization technique. Injuries from these animals are extremely rare and when they bite, they do not always inject venom. However, treat any injuries as genuine life-threatening emergencies. Their injected neurotoxins can rapidly lead to respiratory failure and cardiac arrest. Seek immediate medical attention. Use the following steps if treating an injury by pressure immobilization:

1. Call for help.
2. Place a cloth or gauze pad that measures four inches by four inches (10 cm by 10 cm) by an inch (2.5 cm) thick directly over the wound.
3. Hold the pad in place by wrapping an elastic bandage around the pad and the limb. Wrap at least an inch (2.5 cm) above and below the pad. Wrapping the entire limb is better. Wrap the pad tight enough to press the pad into the skin, but not tight enough to cut off circulation.
4. Apply a splint to immobilize the limb.
5. Monitor the victim for breathing and circulation and signs of an allergic reaction.
6. Transport the victim to medical attention.

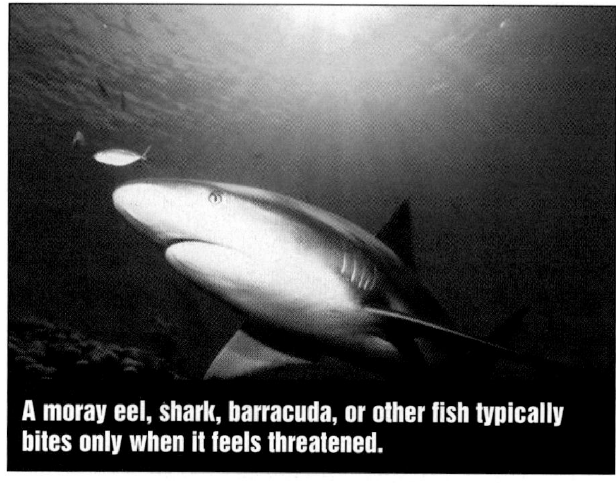

A moray eel, shark, barracuda, or other fish typically bites only when it feels threatened.

BITES

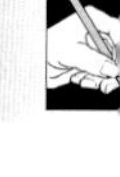

A moray eel, shark, barracuda, or other fish typically bites only when they feel threatened. They can also bite when they are being fed and they miss the bait and get a diver instead. To avoid these situations, always remember to look but don't touch or feed wild animals. Although common in some locales, fish-feeding dives should be avoided. Use the following steps if you see a diver bitten:

1. If the animal is still biting remember that the teeth face inward and although a natural reaction is to pull one's hand away, it may be necessary to unhook by pushing inward first before withdrawing.
2. Assist the diver to the surface.
3. Clean the wound and remove any tooth fragments.
4. Control the bleeding and bandage as necessary.
5. Transport the victim to medical attention for possible stitches and antibiotics, if necessary.

ENVENOMATIONS

Envenomations (injection of venom) occur when you are punctured or stung by an aquatic creature. The types of creatures that can inject venom are:

- Jellyfish
- Sea urchins

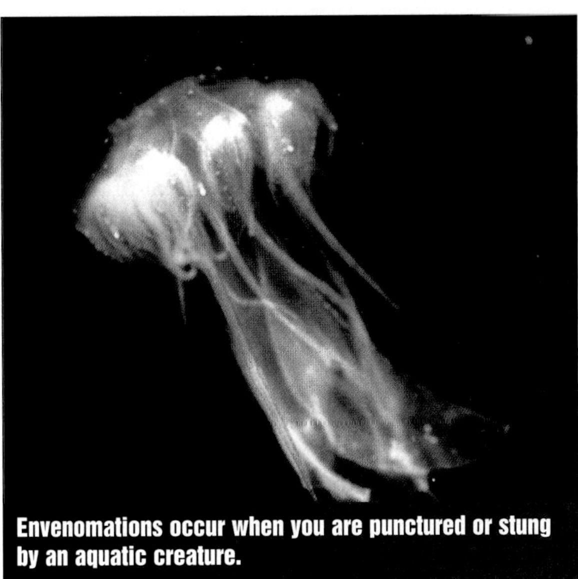

Envenomations occur when you are punctured or stung by an aquatic creature.

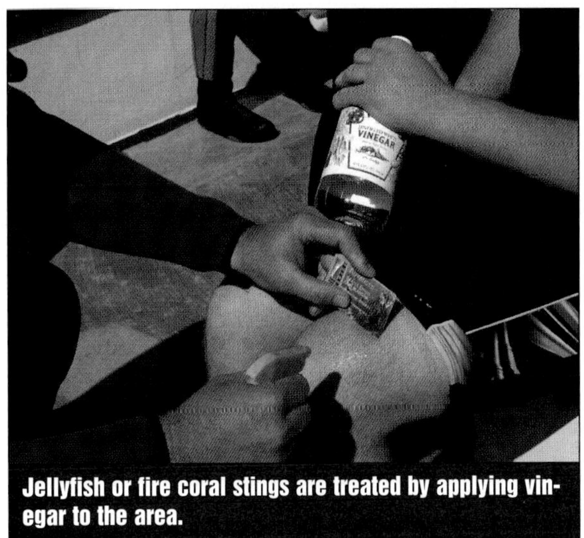

Jellyfish or fire coral stings are treated by applying vinegar to the area.

- Stingrays
- Stonefish, scorpionfish, lionfish, or catfish
- Blue-ringed octopus
- Cone snails (family Conidae)
- Sea snakes
- Bristleworms or fireworms
- Sea cucumbers
- Crown of Thorns seastar
- Sea sponges

Cnidarian (Coelenterate) Stings

Cnidarians or coelenterates include Portuguese man-of-war, fire coral, jellyfish, box jellyfish, sea nettles, hydroids, sea wasps, and anemones. The stinging cells of these creatures are called nematocysts, which inject venom when they come in contact with living tissue (skin).

Coelenterate stings are best prevented by wearing a skin suit that covers you from neck to ankle and has long sleeves. You can also wear gloves to protect your hands.

If you see someone stung, follow the procedure in "Treating by White Vinegar" previously described.

If you see someone stung by a Chironex box jellyfish (found in Australian waters), get help immediately. The lifeguards at many of the beaches in Queensland carry the antivenin needed to counteract a box jellyfish sting. Sea wasps (found in the Caribbean) are also a box jellyfish, but are not as lethal as the Chironex. Their stings also need immediate treatment with hot water, vinegar, and/or papain (an ingredient in papaya juice and meat tenderizers). Monitor the victim for signs of an allergic reaction.

Sea Urchin Puncture

Sea urchins will leave their spines embedded in skin if they are bumped into underwater. The spines can penetrate neoprene wet suits. If you see someone injured by a sea urchin, follow the procedure in "Treating by Heat" previously described.

Then, carefully try to remove the spines. These kinds of spines crumble easily making them hard to remove. Deeply embedded or crumbled spines might need to be removed by medical personnel.

Stingray

Stingrays have a barbed spine in their tail. When they are stepped on, they whip the tail up in the water in a defensive move and strike a leg or foot. When the barb penetrates the skin, venom is injected. If you see someone injured by a stingray, follow the procedure in "Treating by Heat" previously described.

Local lidocane can help with the pain. If the laceration is severe, treat it with first aid and always seek medical attention because delayed problems often occur and the wound may need to be explored.

Fish Spine Envenomations

Stonefish, scorpionfish, and lionfish all have spines and venom in their dorsal fin with which they can stick an unsuspecting diver. These fish blend extremely well with their environment, and a diver can contact one if they are not careful.

Catfish also have spines and venom sacs and will sting if mishandled or provoked. They are found in muddy rivers, lakes, and on beaches in temperate, subtropical, and tropical waters. Both salt- and fresh-water catfish are dangerous.

If you see someone injured by fish spines, follow the procedure in "Treating by Heat" previously described.

Blue-Ringed Octopus Bite

The blue-ringed octopus is a small creature that is sometimes found in tidal pools in Australian and the western Indo-Pacific waters. Do not be fooled by their size. At times, the bite might not be felt and go unnoticed. However, the bite is deadly! The wound is very small and might appear as a blood blister or a small bruise. If you see someone bitten by a blue-ringed octopus, follow the procedure in "Treating by Pressure Immobilization" previously described. Be sure to get the victim to medical attention immediately.

Cone Snail Sting

Cone snails (family Conidae) are pretty to look at but deadly to touch. The cone snail has a proboscis (tubular mouth) at the narrow end of the shell which has a venom-carrying harpoon. The harpoon can penetrate skin and light clothing. If you see someone who has a cone shell puncture, follow the procedure in "Treating by Pressure Immobilization" previously described. Be sure to get the victim to medical attention immediately.

Sea Snake Bite

Sea snakes are found in the tropical and temperate zones in the waters of the Indo-Pacific. You might see a puncture mark at the wound site, but there is little or no pain or inflammation. Often, no venom is injected. However, if venom has been injected, the bite can be deadly. If you see someone bitten by a sea snake, follow the procedure in "Treating by Pressure Immobilization" previously described. Be sure to get the victim to medical attention immediately.

Bristleworms

Bristleworms (or fireworms) are elongated worms with segments. Each segment contains a pair of bristles. The worms live in tropical waters throughout the world. These worms can bite if you handle them or their bristles can penetrate your skin. If you see someone bitten or stung by a bristleworm, follow the procedure in "Treating by White Vinegar" previously described.

Sea Cucumbers

Sea cucumbers have an elongated tubular body. They have tentacles surrounding their mouth. They live in tropical, subtropical, and temperate waters. They are not aggressive, but a rash can occur if you make contact with their excrement or eat a sea cucumber without adequate cooking. If the excrement comes in contact with the eyes, severe eye irritation will occur and can lead to blindness. If you see someone who has come into contact with sea cucumber excrement, follow the procedure in "Treating by White Vinegar" previously described. If the eyes are affected, rinse them with 1 - 2 gallons (4 - 8 liters) of fresh water.

Crown of Thorns Seastar

The Crown of Thorns seastar has as many as 13 - 16 arms. Each arm is covered with spines up to 2 inches (5 centimeters) in length. These sea-stars live in tropical and subtropical waters. Injury occurs when you come in contact with their spines and venom is injected into the wound they cause. If you see someone punctured by a Crown of Thorns seastar spine, follow the procedure in "Treating by Heat" previously described.

Sea Sponges

Sea sponges grow attached to shells, stones, or other solid objects in temperate, subtropical, and tropical waters. Contact by divers is either deliberate or accidental. A widespread rash occurs when you make contact with the spicules of some species of sea sponge. If you see someone who has come in contact with a sea sponge and exhibits a rash or irritation, follow the procedure in "Treating by White Vinegar" previously described.

INGESTED FISH POISONING

Some fish and shellfish are poisonous when you eat them. Cooking or soaking does not destroy many toxins. Also, the fish or shellfish might not taste "off" or smell unusual.

Ciguatera Poisoning

Ciguatera poisoning is the most common form of ingested fish poisoning. Four hundred species of fish are implicated in ciguatera poisoning. They are not all toxic at any one time or in one place. Ciguatera poisoning is sporadic and unpredictable. Some of the species implicated that may cause ciguatera poisoning are:

- Barracuda
- Grouper
- Snapper
- Sea bass
- Surgeonfish
- Mackerel
- Parrotfish
- Wrasse
- Jackfish
- Amberjacks
- Moray eels
- Large reef fish

The signs and symptoms of ciguatera poisoning in the order of most common to least common include:

- Reversal of hot and cold perception
- Chills
- Weakness
- Numbness
- Paresthesias (burning, itching, tingling)
- Arthralgias (joint pain)
- Dizziness
- Diarrhea, nausea, and vomiting
- Abdominal pain

The easiest way to prevent ciguatera poisoning is to avoid eating the fish listed above. Treat all oversized fish with caution as the toxins become more concentrated as they move up through the food chain. Follow the advice of the local inhabitants as you travel throughout the world. If they say you should not eat a certain type of fish in their area, believe them. Use the following steps if you suspect someone has ciguatera poisoning:

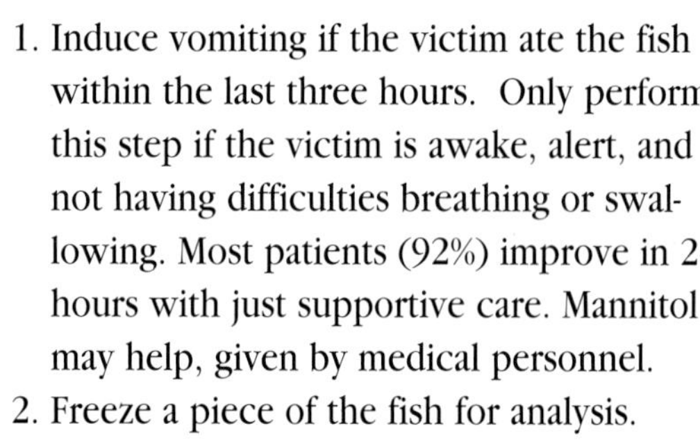

1. Induce vomiting if the victim ate the fish within the last three hours. Only perform this step if the victim is awake, alert, and not having difficulties breathing or swallowing. Most patients (92%) improve in 24 hours with just supportive care. Mannitol may help, given by medical personnel.
2. Freeze a piece of the fish for analysis.
3. Transport the victim to medical attention.

Scombroid Poisoning

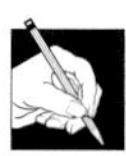

Scombroid poisoning results from eating fish that has not been properly preserved or refrigerated after it is caught. The fish that can cause scombroid poisoning include:

- Albacore, bluefin, and yellowfin tuna
- Mackerel
- Wahoo
- Skipjack
- Bonito
- Bluefish
- Dolphinfish (mahi-mahi)
- Sardines
- Anchovies
- Herring
- Amberjack

The signs and symptoms of scombroid poisoning include:

- Flushed skin of the face, neck, and upper torso that gets worse with exposure to the sun.
- Sensation of warmth without an elevated temperature
- Itching or hives
- Red eyes
- Puffy face and hands
- Difficulty breathing with wheezing
- Nausea, vomiting, and diarrhea
- Headache
- Thirst
- Difficulty swallowing

Prevent scombroid poisoning by eating fish that has been properly refrigerated from the time it is caught. Do not eat any fish that smells of ammonia or has an abnormal taste. Contaminated fish will sometimes have a sharp or peppery flavor. Use the following steps if you suspect someone has scombroid poisoning:

1. Induce vomiting if the victim ate the fish within the last three hours. Only perform this step if the victim is awake, alert, and not having difficulties breathing or swallowing.
2. Transport the victim to medical attention for treatment for an allergic reaction.

Tetrodotoxin Poisoning

Tetrodotoxin poisoning is caused by eating pufferfish, sunfish, or porcupine fish. These fish have a toxin distributed throughout the fish with the highest levels of the toxin in the liver, intestines, gonads, and skin. Specially trained chefs in Japan do prepare a delicacy called Fugu from pufferfish. Nevertheless, about 100 people a year die of Tetrodotoxin poisoning after eating Fugu.

The symptoms of tetrodotoxin poisoning can occur within ten minutes of ingesting the fish, but can be delayed for up to four hours. The signs and symptoms of tetrodotoxin poisoning include:

- Oral numbness and tingling
- Lightheadedness and generalized numbness and tingling
- Drooling
- Difficulty swallowing
- Sweating
- Fatigue
- Headache
- Vomiting, nausea, and diarrhea
- Abdominal pain
- Weakness
- Difficulty walking, incoordination, and uncontrollable shaking
- Paralysis

To avoid tetrodotoxin poisoning, do not eat any fish that does not have scales. If you do eat

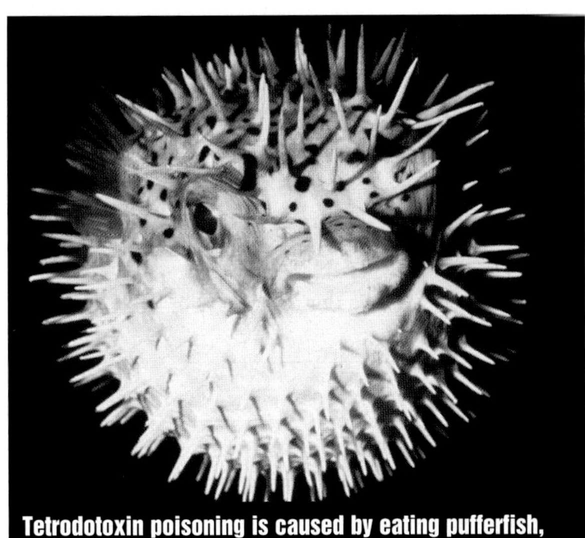

Tetrodotoxin poisoning is caused by eating pufferfish, sunfish, or porcupine fish.

Fugu in Japan or elsewhere, be sure it is prepared by a licensed "puffer" chef. Use the following steps if you suspect someone has tetrodotoxin poisoning:

1. Induce vomiting if the victim ate the fish within the last three hours. Only perform this step if the victim is awake, alert, and not having difficulties breathing or swallowing.
2. Perform artificial respiration if the victim is not breathing.
3. Seek immediate medical attention.

Paralytic Shellfish Poisoning

Paralytic shellfish poisoning is caused by eating shellfish that have ingested large amounts of plankton and protozoans that cause "red tides" or "water blooms." The shellfish concentrate the toxins created by the planktons and protozoans. The shellfish that can cause paralytic shellfish poisoning include:

- Clams
- Oysters
- Scallops
- Mussels

Symptoms of paralytic shellfish poisoning can occur from 20 minutes to many hours after the ingestion of the poison. The signs and symptoms of paralytic shellfish poisoning include:

- Numbness and tingling inside and around the mouth, including the tongue and gums
- Numbness of the neck, hands, and feet
- Weakness
- Floating sensation
- Loss of balance
- Incoordination
- Difficulty speaking and swallowing
- Nausea, vomiting, and diarrhea
- Paralysis

To lessen the effects of paralytic shellfish poisoning, always thoroughly cook shellfish before eating it. If there is an unexplained presence of dead sea creatures in an area, do not eat the shellfish taken from that area. Also, if there is a red tide, do not eat the shellfish. Use the following steps if you suspect someone has paralytic shellfish poisoning:

1. Induce vomiting if the victim ate the shellfish within the last three hours. Only perform this step if the victim is awake, alert, and not having difficulties breathing or swallowing.
2. Perform artificial respiration if the victim is short of breath or unconscious.
3. Reassure the victim. They might be completely paralyzed, but are still conscious and able to hear.
4. Seek immediate medical attention.

REVIEW QUESTIONS

1. Drowning is the ______________________________ of unintended death worldwide following ____, and the leading cause of accidental death of ____.
2. Submersion in cold water can also induce the rapid onset of hypothermia, which has been observed to ____ ____.
3. A barotrauma is ____.
4. You should not ___________ the equalization of your ears ___________________________.
5. Pulmonary barotraumas (lung overexpansion injuries) occur when ___________________ ____.
6. Decompression sickness is caused by inert gas (nitrogen) that has been absorbed into your tissues during a dive ____ ____.
7. Nitrogen narcosis is ______________________________ caused by ___________________ ____.
8. The amount of ___________ needed to trigger seasickness ___________________________ ____.
9. Wounds in the aquatic environment are contaminated with ___________________________ ____, and other organic matter.
10. Many toxins are heat labile, meaning____.
11. Aquatic injuries caused by stinging cells (nematocysts) of jellyfish, fire coral, and so on are treated with ____ to neutralize the toxin.
12. Bites from a blue-ringed octopus or a sea snake, or a puncture from a cone shell are treated with ____.
13. A moray eel, shark, barracuda, or other fish typically bites only when _________________ ____.

14. The types of creatures that can inject venom are: - list 6 of the 11 creatures from the text.

____

____

____

____

____

____

15. Ciguatera poisoning is ______________________________

______________________________.

16. Scombroid poisoning results from eating fish ______________________________

______________________________.

17. Tetrodotoxin poisoning is caused by eating ______________________________

______________________________.

18. Paralytic shellfish poisoning is caused by eating ______________ that have ingested large amounts of plankton and protozoans that cause ______________________________ .

CHAPTER 18

Moving and Transporting Victims

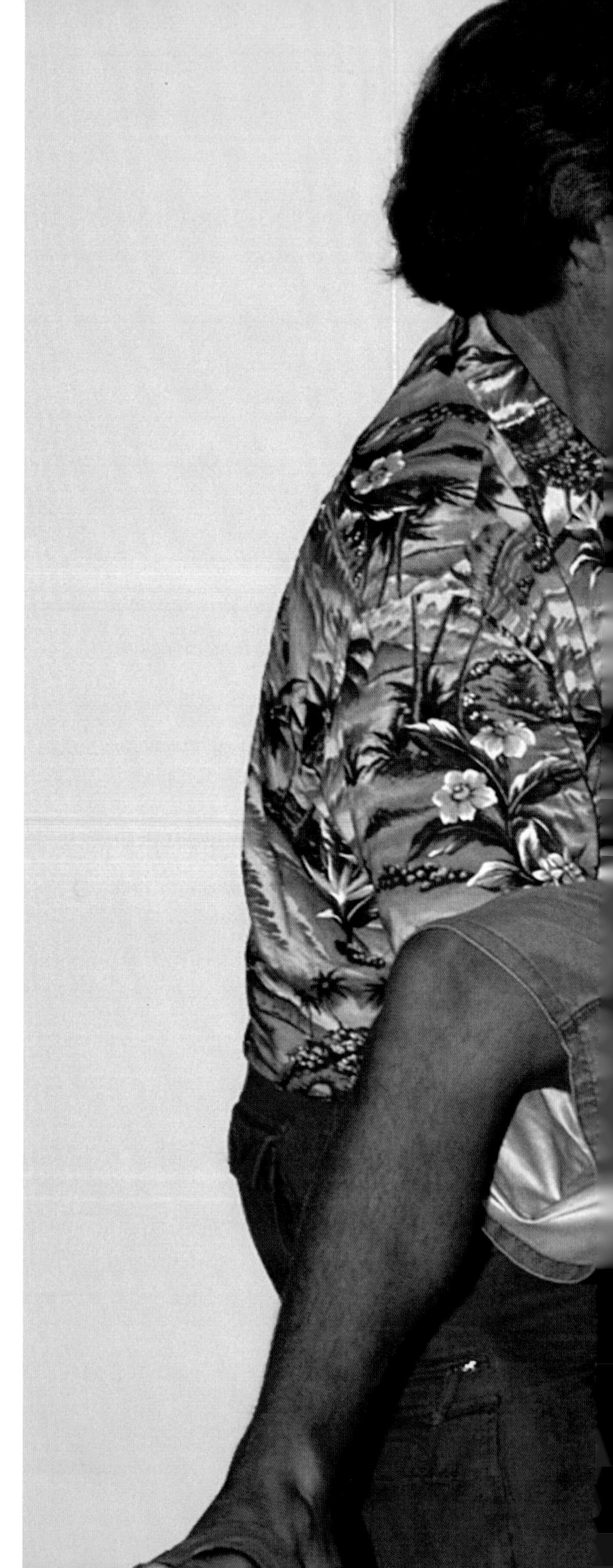

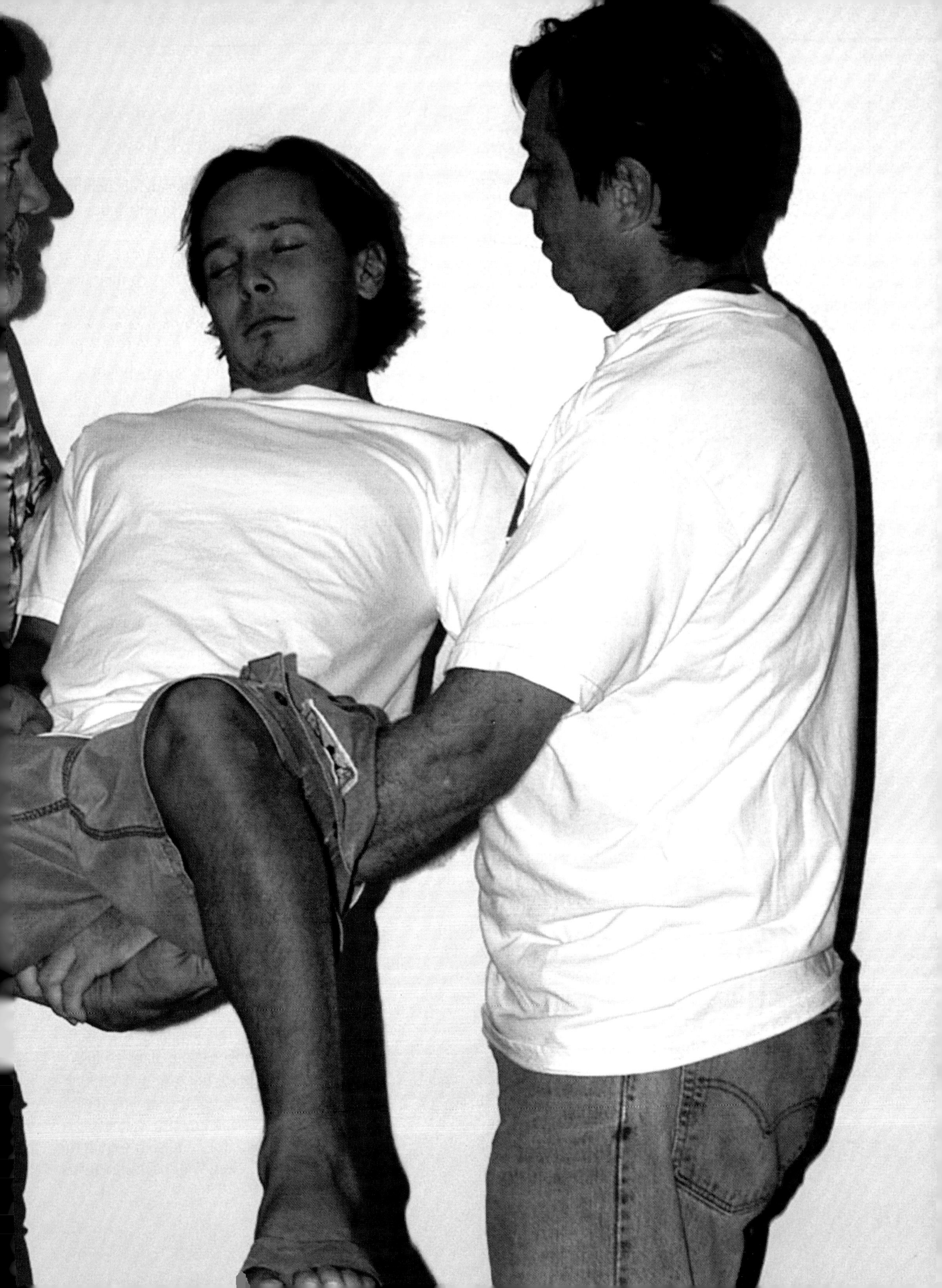

MOVING AND TRANSPORTING VICTIMS

(Moving and transporting victims in the water and removing them from the water are covered in NAUI's Rescue Scuba Diver textbook.)

LEARNING GOALS

In this chapter you will learn about:

- Considerations for moving a victim
- Clothes and underarm drag
- Firefighter's carry
- Packstrap carry
- Two-person carry
- Three- or more-person carry
- Walking assist
- Litter or Backboard carry

Your primary concern if you need to move a victim is to do no further harm. You should only move a victim if you find yourself in one of the following situations:

- There is an immediate danger to the victim such as fire, explosion, a collapsing structure, lack of oxygen, or other immediate threats to the victim's safety.
- You need to get to another victim who is more seriously hurt, and the first victim is in the way.
- You need to move the victim to be able to provide proper care, such as a victim in the water or under a collapsed structure.

There are a number of ways to move a victim. The method you choose depends on the size of the victim and your size, the extent of injury to the victim, and whether you have help.

CLOTHES DRAG

This is a good method to move a conscious or unconscious victim if the victim cannot walk and you are alone. You should also use this method if you suspect a neck or spinal injury. Use the following steps to move the victim:

1. Gather the victim's clothes tightly behind the victim's neck, without constricting their airway.
2. Use the clothes and your hands to support the victim's neck to better keep their head, neck, and spine aligned.
3. Pull the clothes to move the victim. When attempting this drag, be sure to bend at your knees with your torso as upright as possible to avoid bending over and to ensure a proper lifting posture, then lean back in the direction of the drag so that gravity and your leg muscles do the work.

UNDER-ARM DRAG

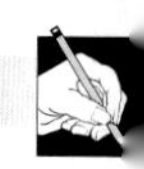

This is an alternative carry to the clothes drag. Use the following steps for an under-arm drag:

1. Stand behind the victim.
2. Place your hands under the victim's armpits.
3. Use your upper arms to cradle the victim's neck and head.
4. When attempting this drag, be sure to bend at your knees with your torso as upright as possible to avoid bending over and to ensure a proper lifting posture, then lean back in the direction of the drag so that gravity and your leg muscles do the work.

FIREFIGHTER'S CARRY

A firefighter's carry can be used if the rescuer is strong enough and the victim is not too large. It is a good method to use if you need to move a conscious or unconscious victim quickly and you do not suspect a neck or spinal injury. Use the following steps to move the victim:

1. If the victim is unconscious stand facing the victim and place the front half of your feet on the front half of the victim's feet
2. Bend your knees and grab the victim's wrists. Lean backward and start to pull the victim upright. Keep your back straight as

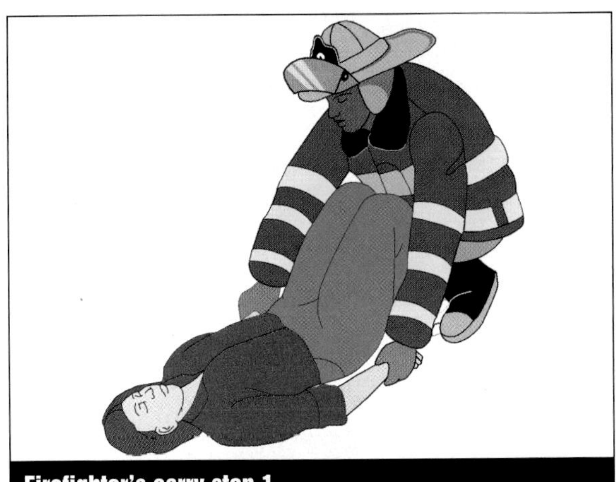

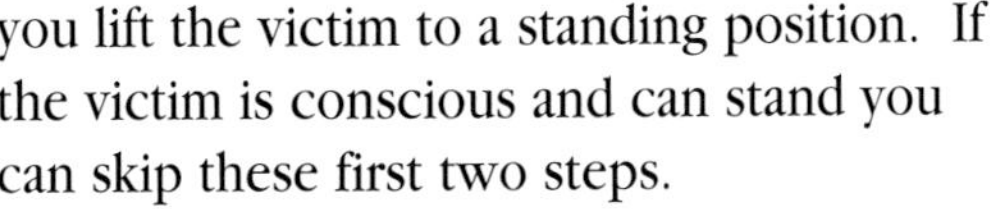

Firefighter's carry step 1

you lift the victim to a standing position. If the victim is conscious and can stand you can skip these first two steps.

3. Release one of their wrists and pivot to the side while pulling with the other hand so that the victim begins to lean over you as you quickly bend your knees and duck your shoulder under the victim's torso.
4. Position the victim so that the bulk of their weight rests across your shoulders and your free hand can reach between their legs at the crotch.
5. Use your legs to stand up and complete the lift.
6. Walk until you have reached safety.

PACKSTRAP CARRY

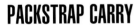

This is a good method to use if you need to move a conscious or unconscious victim quickly and you do not suspect a neck or spinal injury. Use the following steps to move the victim:

1. Position the victim on their back with their knees bent in a 90-degree angle.
2. Stand facing the victim and place the front half of your feet on the front half of the victim's feet.
3. Bend your knees and grab the victim's right wrist with your right hand and the victim's left wrist with your left hand forming an "X" with your forearms.

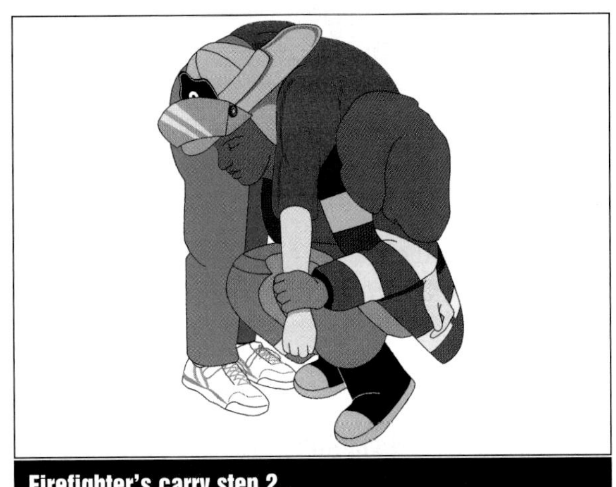

Firefighter's carry step 2

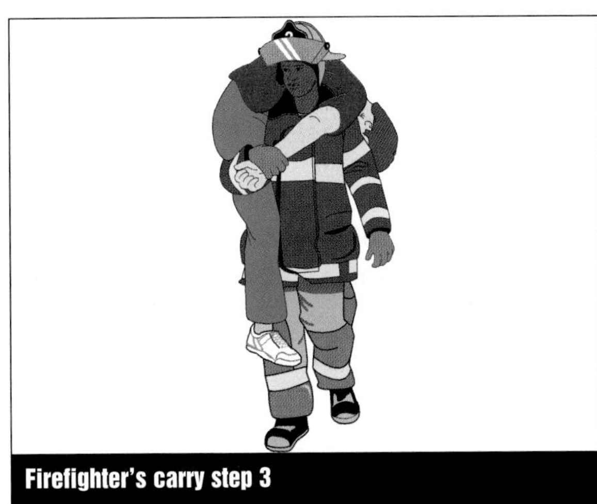

Firefighter's carry step 3

4. Lean backward and start to pull the victim upright. Keep your back straight as you lift the victim.
5. Pivot in the direction of your top arm as the victim approaches the upright position.
6. Continue pivoting until you have turned 180 degrees and lift the victim's arms over your shoulders and cross them to form an X. By holding the wrist of the victim's top arm you can free your other arm to steady yourself.
7. Lean forward, pulling forward and down on the victim's arms until their feet are off the ground, positioning the victim's armpits on the top of your shoulders.
8. Walk until you have reached safety.

TWO-PERSON CARRY

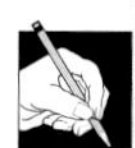

This is a good method to use if the victim is conscious but cannot walk, and you have assistance. Use the following steps for the two-person carry:

1. Face the other rescuer and interlock your arms (hold on to each other's wrists or forearms).
2. Put one set of arms behind the victim's back and the other set under the victim's thighs.
3. Lift the seated victim by using your legs to lift.

THREE- OR MORE-PERSON CARRY

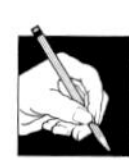

This is a good method to use if the victim is unconscious, you don't have a litter or backboard, and you have assistance. Use the following steps for the three-person carry:

1. Divide your group so that you can lift the victim from both sides. Rescuers should be staggered rather than facing each other directly across the victim.
2. Position the victim on their back.
3. Kneel (on the knee closest to the victim's feet) next to the victim, facing the victim, and side by side (if you have a partner).
4. Reach across and above the victim to locate arm position so that each rescuer is grasping the wrist of each of their alternates, right to right and so on.
5. The rescuer at the victim's head must support the head and neck so that they remain aligned with the spine throughout the lift and transport. This rescuer also acts as a leader and signals when to lift and when to carry.(It is also a good idea to place the strongest rescuers at the head and torso of the victim.)
6. Reach under the victim and grasp your alternates' wrists.
7. On a signal from the leader, everyone lifts at once keeping their back straight and lifting with their legs until the victim is at the knee height - the victim's weight can be supported on the raised knee and thigh. When everyone has re-secured their grip the leader can signal all to stand. This two phase lift allows more control and is easier for the weaker members of the team.
8. When everyone is ready, the leader can signal for transport so that everyone begins walking at one time.

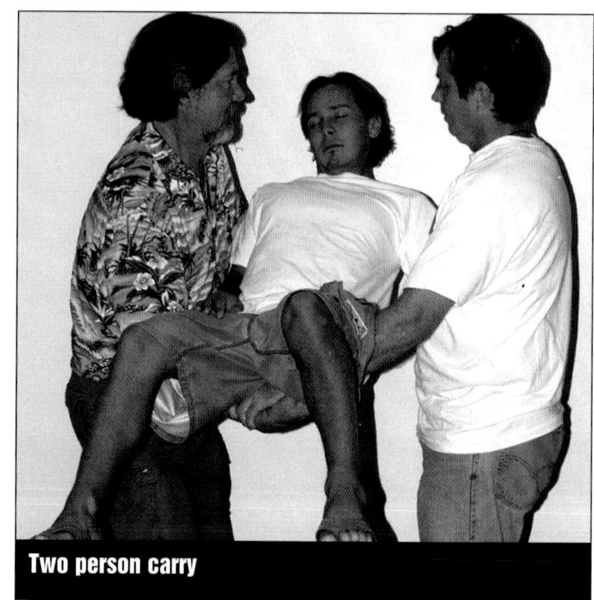
Two person carry

WALKING ASSIST

This is a good method to use if the victim can walk with assistance. You can use this assist alone or when you have help. Use the following steps for the walking assist:

1. Place the victim's arm over your shoulder.
2. Hold the arm in place with your hand.
3. Support the victim with your other arm around their waist to help them walk. If you have assistance, they can support the victim on the other side.

LITTER OR BACKBOARD CARRY

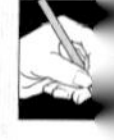

You should use this carry only if you have at least four adults to help or the victim is small enough that fewer people can lift the litter or backboard. The litter or backboard must be extremely firm and not subject to bending if the injured person has a suspected neck or back injury. Otherwise, a flexible litter will work, for example a hammock, a sling chair, and many bamboo carriers common in Asia. You must know how to tie some basic knots to be able to tie the victim to the litter. Use the following steps for the backboard carry:

1. Keep one rescuer at the head of the victim at all times, holding the neck immobile with gentle but firm pressure.
2. Roll the victim onto their side, keeping their head and back in a straight line.
3. Place the litter against the victim's back.
4. Roll the victim back onto the litter, while still stabilizing the head and neck.
5. Make sure that the victim is horizontally centered on the litter and that no part of their body is off the litter at the top or bottom.
6. Gather four ties (triangular bandage, strips of linen, etc.). Each piece should be at least 6 feet (2 meters) long.
7. Tie the victim to the litter, starting with the legs, then the pelvis, then the chest, and finally the forehead.
8. Place padding into any spaces between the ties, the litter, and the victim to aid in immobilization and comfort.
9. Place padding under the buttocks and heels, but only enough to prevent pressure during transport, not enough to change positioning, or move the spine.
10. Cover the victim to keep them comfortably warm.
11. Position one rescuer at the head of the litter to serve as the leader.
12. Position the other rescuers at the foot of and along the sides of the litter, with at least one resucer on each side.
13. Have each rescuer grasp the litter with one hand.
14. Lift on the leader's call, keeping your back straight.

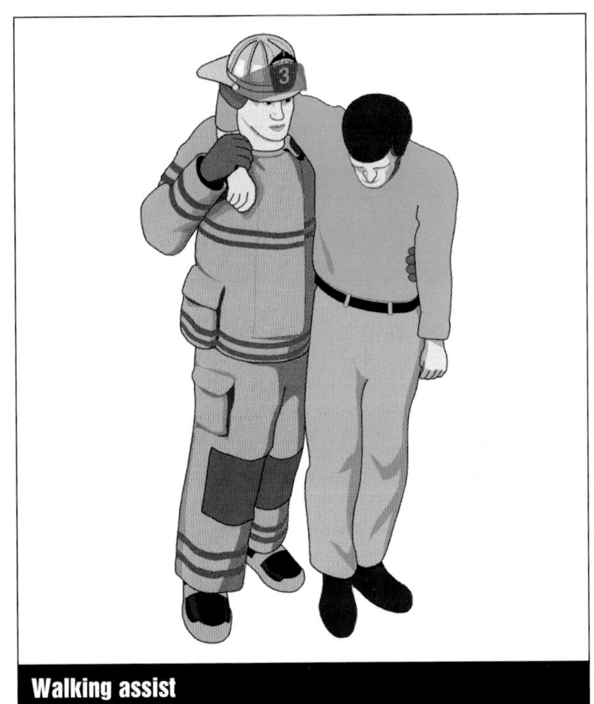

Walking assist

15. Adjust each rescuer's lifting height as necessary to keep the victim level.
16. At the leader's call the other rescuers support the litter while the leader turns around.
17. Move on the leader's call. The leader should start off with his left foot while all the others start of with their right foot. This will prevent the litter from swinging side-to-side during transport.
18. Walk as far as you can before resting. The leader should be looking ahead for dangers and obstacles.
19. Stop when necessary to monitor injuries, re-secure knots, readjust padding, or rest.

REVIEW QUESTIONS

1. Your primary concern if you need to move a victim is ______________________________ ____.
2. The __________________ is a good method to move a conscious or unconscious victim if the victim cannot walk and you are alone.
3. The __________________ is an alternative carry to the clothes drag.
4. A firefighter's carry can be used if the rescuer is ______________ and the victim is ____.
5. The ____________________is a good method to use if you need to move a conscious or unconscious victim quickly and you do not suspect a neck or spinal injury.
6. The __________________________is a good method to use if the victim is conscious but cannot walk, and you have assistance.
7. The _________________________ is a good method to use if the victim is unconscious, you don't have a litter or backboard, and you have assistance.
8. You should use the Litter or Backboard Carry only if you have at least ______ adults to help or the victim is ____ ____..

Notes